REGULATING
INFANT
FORMULA

GEORGE KENT

Regulating Infant Formula

George Kent
Department of Political Science
University of Hawai'i

Hale Publishing, L.P.

1712 N. Forest St.

Amarillo, TX 79106-7017

806-376-9900

800-378-1317

www.iBreastfeeding.com

Library of Congress Control Number: 2011939924

ISBN-13: 978-0-9833075-8-7

Printing and Binding: Corley Printing Company

Acknowledgments

It is with deep gratitude that I acknowledge the generous advice of James Akre, Carol Bartle, Stephen Buescher, Ted Greiner, Arly Helm, Louise James, Maureen Minchin, Pamela Morrison, Touraj Shafai, Julie Smith, Virginia Thorley, Marian Tompson, and Margret Vidar during the preparation of this book.

Dedication

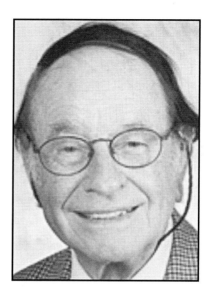

This book is dedicated to the late Michael Latham, a wonderful champion of optimum infant feeding and mentor to many students and colleagues. He was memorialized by the New York Times on April 13, 2011, at http://www.nytimes. com/2011/04/14/health/14latham.html?_r=2.

Table of Contents

Introduction

The choice of infant feeding methods impacts the child, the family, and the broader society on many dimensions. While the benefits and risks to children's health with different feeding methods are relatively clear, there are other factors to be considered.

The major benefits of feeding with formula are related not to the child's direct interests, but rather to the family's interests. Under some conditions, using infant formula may be a prudent choice, even though it involves some risk to the infant's wellbeing (Dorfman, 2010).

Advertising and other forms of promotion, and government programs that insulate their participants from the cost of formula and from healthcare costs can lead families to make unwise decisions. Parents do not get the information they need in order to make properly informed choices. This book is about governments' obligations to prevent children from being exposed to excessive risk due to the use of infant formula.

Marion Nestle (not related to the similarly named company) describes the context:

> Infant formulas are flashpoints for contention for three important reasons: they are largely unnecessary (most mothers can breastfeed their infants), are less perfect than breast-

milk for feeding babies, and are more expensive than breastfeeding. Breast-milk is nutritionally superior to formula, but from a marketing standpoint, it has one serious disadvantage: it is free. Beyond one-time purchases of breast pumps, storage bottles, or special clothing, nobody makes money from it.

For mothers who cannot, should not, or do not want to breastfeed, formula is a socially and nutritionally acceptable substitute. But formula companies do not only promote formulas to mothers who must use formula. In subtle and not-so-subtle ways, they promote the use of formulas to all pregnant women and new mothers (Nestle, 2006, p. 452).

Based on her observations in low-income countries, pediatrician Cicely Williams first raised alarm about the impact of artificial feeding publicly in a speech in 1939 entitled "Milk and Murder." Her conclusion did not mince words:

If you are legal purists, you may wish me to change the title of this address to Milk and Manslaughter. But if your lives were embittered as mine is, by seeing day after day this massacre of the innocents by unsuitable feeding, then I believe you would feel as I do that misguided propaganda on infant feeding should be punished as the most criminal form of sedition, and that these deaths should be regarded as murder (Baumslag, 2006, pp. 58-62).

Sweetened condensed milk was in widespread use at that time, especially in Asia. Infant formulas are no longer made with condensed or evaporated milks. They have steadily improved, but there is still excessive mortality and morbidity associated with their use. There is now an emerging recognition that the problems are not entirely due to poor living conditions. The excessive mortality and morbidity associated with the use of infant formula in high-income countries shows that the problems are due in part to the infant formula itself.

Others have examined the infant formula industry from various angles. For example, Judith Richter focused on the industry in her book, *Holding Corporations Accountable* (Richter, 2001). The International Baby Food Action Network regularly scrutinizes the performance of corporations in terms of the standards set out in the *International Code of Marketing of Breast-Milk Substitutes*, and examines the degree to which national governments include the Code in their national law and act to implement it. The perspective of this book is that not only corporations, but also governments need to be held accountable for a broad range of issues relating to infant formula. We usually view governments as the regulators, but they, too, need to be watched.

The manufacturers of infant formula are under pressure to maximize their profits. The premise here is that the primary interest of government agencies responsible for the regulation of food for infants and young children should be the health and wellbeing of the children and their mothers, in the short term and the long term. Others' interests may be served in some measure, but that should not be done in ways that put children at significant risk.

This book shows that government regulation of the manufacture and marketing of infant formula is flawed in many ways. These are not random flaws. The regulatory process is skewed in favor of private economic interests, especially those of infant formula manufacturers. This skew is at the expense of infants, exposing them to excessive risks.

1 The Regulatory Framework

At the global level, the *Codex Alimentarius Commission* develops non-binding guidelines regarding food composition and safety, including infant formula. The Food and Agriculture Organization of the United Nations and the World Health Organization jointly established the Commission in 1963. Its main purposes are "protecting health of the consumers and ensuring fair trade practices in the food trade, and promoting coordination of all food standards work undertaken by international governmental and non-governmental organizations" (Codex Alimentarius Commission, 2011, para 1). It does this by developing food standards, guidelines, and related texts, such as codes of practice under the Joint FAO/WHO Food Standards Program.

In 1976, at its 11th session, the Codex Alimentarius Commission issued a *Statement on Infant Feeding*. It said, "it is necessary to encourage breastfeeding by all possible means in order to prevent that the decline in breastfeeding, which seems to be actually occurring, does not lead to artificial methods of infant feeding which could be inadequate or could have an adverse effect on the health of the infant" (Codex Alimentarius Commission, 1976, para 4).

At this session in 1976, the Commission also adopted a *Codex Standard for Infant Formula*. The standard, designated as CODEX STAN 72-1981, includes a list of required ingredients and names various required quality control measures. In 1983, the 15th Session adopted amendments to the sections on Food Additives and Labeling. A further amendment to the Labeling section was adopted in 1985 by the 16th Session. Amendments to the Vitamin D and B12 amounts were adopted by the 17th (1987) and 22nd (1997) Sessions, respectively (Codex Alimentarius Commission, 2007).

This core statement of the required ingredients for infant formula is generally accepted throughout the world. The permitted nutrient ranges legitimized a broad variety of quite different existing formulas. The requirements are widely regarded as a minimum standard. Some high-income countries have adopted more stringent requirements.

In 1979 Codex issued *Advisory Lists of Mineral Salts and Vitamin Compounds for use in Foods for Infants and Children*, and revised these lists in 1983 and 1991. In 2001 it issued a statement on maximum levels of lead in a broad variety of foods, including infant formula. Other modifications have been discussed, but the Codex standard for infant formula remains much the same as that published in 1981.

Codex has a *Code of Hygienic Practice for Powdered Formulae for Infants and Young Children,* last updated in 2008 (Codex Alimentarius Commission, 2008).

In addition to the guidelines provided by *Codex Alimentarius,* there is another set of global guidelines. Steadily growing concern over the ways in which the use of commercial infant formula has been promoted led to the adoption of the *International Code of Marketing of Breast-Milk Substitutes* by the World Health Assembly on May 21, 1981. Subsequent resolutions of the World Health Assembly help to clarify and extend the Code (Latham, 1997; Richter, 2001; Shubber, 1998; Shubber, 2011; World Health Organization, 1981). A strong global network of non-governmental organizations, the International Baby Food Action Network, emerged to help ensure the implementation of the Code (IBFAN, 2011).

As stated in its first article:

> The aim of this Code is to contribute to the provision of safe and adequate nutrition for infants, by the protection and promotion of breast-feeding, and by ensuring the proper use of breast-milk substitutes, when these are necessary, on the basis of adequate information and through appropriate marketing and distribution (p. 8).

The second article explains the scope of application of the Code:

> The Code applies to the marketing, and practices related thereto, of the following products: breast-milk substitutes, including infant formula; other milk products, foods and beverages, including bottlefed complementary foods, when marketed or otherwise represented to be suitable, with or without modification, for use as a partial or total replacement of breast-milk; feeding bottles and teats. It also applies to their quality and availability, and to information concerning their use (p. 8).

The Code interprets marketing broadly, as product promotion, distribution, selling, advertising, product public relations, and information services.

The Executive Board of the United Nation's Children's Fund endorsed the Code a few months after its adoption in 1981.

In the European Union, infant formula regulations are set out in "Commission Directive 2006/141/EC of 22 December 2006 on infant formulae and follow-on formulae and amending Directive 1999/21/EC" (EUR-Lex, 2011). It follows the *Codex Alimentarius* guidelines, including its list of required ingredients for infant formula. The Commission Directive also affirms support of the *International Code of Marketing of Breast-Milk Substitutes*:

In an effort to provide better protection for the health of infants, the rules of composition, labeling and advertising laid down in this Directive should be in conformity with the principles and the aims of the *International Code of Marketing of Breast-milk Substitutes* adopted by the 34th World Health Assembly, bearing in mind the particular legal and factual situations existing in the Community (EUR-Lex, 2011, para 27 & Article 1 para 2).

While there is this language supporting the Code in the Commission Directive, IBFAN judges that the language of the Directive and the performance of the countries do not adequately support the Code (IBFAN, 2009a, 2009b).

The Food and Drug Administration (FDA) and the United States Department of Agriculture (USDA) share jurisdiction over food issues in the U.S., but foods specifically for children are under the FDA. The Federal Food, Drug, and Cosmetic Act defines infant formula in Title 21, Section 321(z) of the United States Code. It is "a food that purports to be or is represented for special dietary use solely as a food for infants by reason of its simulation of human milk or its suitability as a complete or partial substitute for human milk" (21 U.S. Code 321 (z).

Section 350a of the act provides specifications regarding adulteration, quality factor requirements, manufacturing regulations, product testing, and record keeping. It sets out a list of required nutrients and their minimum and maximum quantities. The list includes protein, fat, essential fatty acids (only linoleate is in the list), fifteen different vitamins, and eleven different minerals. The list conforms to the recommendations of *Codex Alimentarius*.

The *U.S. Code of Federal Regulations Title 21, Part 106*, specifies infant formula quality control procedures. Last revised in 2009, it is mainly about quality control during the manufacturing process, and not directly about quality of the product that emerges from that process (U.S. Code of Federal Regulations (21CFR106), 2009).

Part 107, last revised in 2003, states the nutrient requirements and other rules regarding labeling, recalls, etc. (U.S. Code of Federal Regulations (21CFR107), 2003).

U.S. rules have been summarized as follows:

> Infant formula, like no other food, is regulated by its own law, the Infant Formula Act of 1980 as amended in 1986. The act sets lower limits on 29 nutrients (so called "table nutrients" because they appear in table form. U.S. Code of Federal Regulations 21 CFR 107.100). . . Manufacturers are required to follow "good manufacturing practice," but no requirement for sterility is specified. . . . Powdered formula is not guaranteed nor required to be free of pathogenic organisms (Baker, 2002, para 3).

The *International Code of Marketing of Breast-Milk Substitutes* is not recognized in U.S. law, but the Code has been used as a basis for critically assessing the ways in which infant formula is promoted in the U.S. (Walker, 2001, 2007).

The U.S. Food and Drug Administration describes U.S. policy and regulations in a consumer-oriented primer, *FDA 101: Infant Formula,* and also in *Infant Formula – Q&A* (U.S. Department of Health and Human Services, 2011c, 2011e).

A good account of the system of regulation in the United Kingdom may be found in Helen Crawley and Susan Westland's *Infant Milks in the UK* (Crawley & Westland, 2011; also see NCT, 2008; NCT, 2010). Australia and New Zealand's regulations are summarized in its *Regulatory Impact Statement* (Australia, 2011). Many countries have adapted the *International Code of Marketing of Breast-Milk Substitutes*, at least to some degree, as documented by the International Baby Food Action Network. Information on the legal and institutional framework for dealing with infant feeding issues in many other countries can be found by searching through the Internet.

Many countries either have no specific regulations regarding infant formula or adopt regulations that generally follow the *Codex Alimentarius* guidelines and the *International Code of Marketing of Breast-Milk Substitutes*. Together, these two establish the global framework for regulation of infant formula.

Thus, there is a layered system of regulation, with guidelines from the global level, and binding regional regulations in Europe. Worldwide, most binding regulation is at the national level. In some large countries, there may be additional sub-national regulations in states and provinces, and in some cases, there may be city-level regulations as well. The rules in large programs that deal with infant and young child feeding, such as those in hospitals and social service programs, also can be viewed as part of the regulatory framework. Given the scope and diversity of these different sets of regulations for infant formula, and their uneven implementation, this book can only offer a broad overview.

The next ten chapters highlight issues that require deeper attention by all agencies that influence the ways in which infant formula is manufactured, marketed, and used.

2 Formula's Impacts on Health

In terms of health considerations, there are few conditions under which children should not be breastfed by their biological mothers or, where necessary, by another woman. According to a study commissioned by the U.S. government, there are no nutritional contraindications to breastfeeding infants, except for infants with inherited disorders, such as galactosemia. The general recommendation is that breast-milk should not be withheld from any infant unless absolutely necessary (Lawrence & Lawrence, 2011). Breastfeeding is not recommended when the mother has certain infectious diseases, has taken certain medications or street drugs, or has certain contaminants in her breast-milk (Hale, 2010). The American Academy of Pediatrics says, "Pediatricians and other healthcare professionals should recommend human milk for all infants in whom breastfeeding is not specifically contraindicated ..." (American Academy of Pediatrics, 2005, p. 498). There is an ongoing discussion of risks relating to breastfeeding at http://www.infantrisk.com/.

Premature infants and infants with disabilities might not be able to breast *feed*, but nevertheless many can use breast *milk*, whether from their own mothers or from donors. For infants who are unable to breastfeed directly from their mothers, the best alternatives are using the mother's own expressed milk or donor milk from another woman, which may need to be pasteurized or heat-treated.

Probably less than one percent of infants need to use infant formula for medical reasons. Apart from infants' health requirements, some needs of parents might make the use of infant formula sensible for a segment of the population.

This book is not about special infant formula for infants with unusual needs, but about commercial infant formula of the sort used by generally healthy infants and mothers. The question is, in dealing with a population, what kinds of public policy would help to protect infants from excessive risks related to the choice of feeding methods?

Some people speak about the benefits of breastfeeding. However, the perspective adopted here is that breastfeeding is the norm, the gold standard against which other methods of infant feeding should be assessed (Akre, 2006; McNiel, Labbok, & Abrahams, 2010; Wiessinger, 1996).

The American Academy of Pediatrics is explicit about this: "Exclusive breastfeeding is the reference or normative model against which all alternative feeding methods must be measured with regard to growth, health, development, and all other short- and long-term outcomes" (American Academy of Pediatrics, 2005, p. 496). Yet few studies offer comparisons of the health impacts of infant formula with the health impacts of exclusive breastfeeding.

All types of impacts, short term and long term, should be assessed and taken into account in choosing methods of feeding. Making objective information about these impacts available to parents in suitable forms is primarily the responsibility of governments.

Many studies have demonstrated the linkages between infant feeding patterns and their morbidity and mortality. In one study in Brazil, "infants who received powdered milk or cow's milk, in addition to breast-milk, were at 4.2 times ... the risk of death from diarrhea compared with infants who did not receive artificial milk, while the risk for infants who did not receive any breast-milk was 14.2 times higher .... Similar results were obtained when infants who died from diarrhea were compared with infants who died from diseases that were presumed to be due to noninfectious causes" (Victora et al., 1989, p. 1032).

A study in the U.S. in 1910 found that bottle-fed infants were six times more likely to die than breastfed ones. Between 1911 and 1916, additional studies showed the same six-fold increase in risk for poorer families, and a four-fold increase in risk for richer families (Richter, 2001).

The use of infant formula tends to increase children's morbidity and mortality, and it has adverse effects on their physical and mental development (Akre, 2009, p. 4; Bartick & Reinhold, 2010; Chen & Rogan, 2004; Fewtrell, 2004; Goldberg, Prentice, Prentice, Filteau, & Simondon, 2009; Lawrence & Lawrence, 2011; Labbok, Clark, & Goldman, 2004; León-Cava, Lutter, Ross, & Martin, 2002; McNiel et al., 2010; Minchin, 1998a, 1998b; Oddy, 2002; Packard, 1982; Palmer, 2009; Smith & Harvey, 2011; U.S. Department of Health and Human Services, 2011a; Wolf, 2003; World Health Organization, 2007a). It has been estimated that, worldwide, if every infant was exclusively breastfed from birth for six months, more than a million lives could be saved each year (UNICEF, 2004).

Many more references, testimonials, and rants in support of breastfeeding may be found at http://www.whale.to/w/baby_milk.html. This source should be used with care because of the uneven credibility of the entries.

The choice of feeding methods has health consequences, not only for the child, but also for the mother (Akre, 2009, p. 4). For example, it has been shown that breastfeeding reduces the incidence of breast cancer (World Cancer, 2007). The U.S. government's National Women's Health Information Center identifies the major benefits of breastfeeding for children in terms of nutrition and growth benefits, and also enhanced immune systems and resistance to infection. It also describes the health benefits for the mother (U.S. Department of Health and Human Services, 2004b). The American Dietetic Association provides similar information on the health benefits of breastfeeding to both the child and the mother (American Dietetic Association, 2001).

Many people believe there is no reason for hesitation in using infant formula. National governments allow it to be sold, and sometimes provide it directly. Many people are confident that their governments are watchful and actively ensure the safety and effectiveness of the product. Thus, it is important to determine whether the standards used by governments to assess formula really are adequate.

The United States government regulates infant formula, but, nevertheless, formula feeding in the U.S. leads to substantial numbers of excess infant deaths. According to a study published in 2004, the risk of postneonatal (29-365 days of age) mortality is about 27 percent higher among infants who are never breastfed compared to infants who are ever breastfed. On this basis, about 720 infant deaths in the U.S. would be averted each year if all infants were breastfed (Chen & Rogan, 2004).

The impact on mortality of not breastfeeding probably was understated. First, the study excluded neonatal deaths (0-28 days), which means that infants who died of necrotizing enterocolitis (NEC) were not counted. These deaths are far more common in formula-fed infants than in breastfed infants. Second, "because exposure to breastfeeding was categorized based on the infant ever being breastfed, the estimate is based on a mixture of breastfeeding exposure levels, including many who were breastfed for a very brief period" (Nommsen-Rivers, 2004, p. 358). Thus, "the estimate of 720 lives saved is likely to be an underestimate compared to the additional effect of continued breastfeeding" (Nommsen-Rivers, 2004, p. 358). If the study had examined exclusively breastfed infants, their mortality rate probably would have been lower than the rates for those that mixed breastfeeding and formula feeding. Third, if deaths beyond the first year were included, the estimate for the number of deaths associated with not breastfeeding would be higher.

Another study, published in 2010, estimated, "If 90% of US families could comply with medical recommendations to breastfeed exclusively for six months, the United States would ... prevent an excess of 911 deaths, nearly all of which would be in infants . . ." (Bartick & Reinhold, 2010, p. e1048).

A few letters to the *Pediatrics* journal raised questions about the methodology used in the Bartick study, with some saying it underestimated the harm done by suboptimal infant feeding. The exact numerical conclusions of this and similar studies are open to dispute. Some skeptics raise questions about the entire body of research relating to infant feeding and say the science in support of breastfeeding is weak (Fentiman, 2010, p. 22; Rosin, 2009). However, the weight of evidence is clear: when compared with breastfeeding, the use of infant formula in the general population results in increased mortality and morbidity, and increased healthcare and other costs.

Apart from the higher mortality, there are many children's illnesses that occur at higher rates as a result of not breastfeeding. In both high-income and low-income countries, the consequences of not breastfeeding are more likely to show up as increased likelihood of illness rather than death.

Most studies on the impacts of infant feeding methods have focused on short-term effects on morbidity (illness) and mortality (death), especially in low-income settings. However, the choice of feeding methods affects infants' health, not only in the short term, but also in the long term, into their adult years (Fewtrell, 2004; Horwood & Fergusson, 1998; Stanner & Smith, 2005; U.S. Department of Health and Human Services, 2011b; Whitehouse, Robinson, Li, & Oddy, 2011; World Health Organization, 2007a). Some types of malnutrition even have intergenerational effects, so it is possible that some of the impacts affect children not only into their adult years, but also affect their children. Thus, studies that assess only short-term impacts underestimate the total harm that results from formula feeding.

Diets have important impacts, not only on morbidity and mortality, but also on physical, reproductive, and mental development. Such long-term problems can be detected only through analysis of statistical patterns at the population level. For example, the dangers associated with trans-fats (partially hydrogenated oils) are detected not through examination of specific events, but of broad patterns: did people who ate more of this type of food have more of these types of consequences? Outcomes, such as cancers, clogged arteries, excessive body weight, or cognitive disorders, are tied not to specific food items, but to dietary patterns.

Historically, much of the criticism of infant formula has focused on short-term problems in low-income countries. This was sensible because there has been far more morbidity and mortality resulting from formula use in low-income than in high-income countries. This led many people to believe that the problems were mainly due to issues such as poor sanitation and low literacy levels. However, it is now being recognized that formula feeding in *any* population leads to worse health consequences for children. This means the problems are not only about deficiencies in the living conditions; they are also about deficiencies in the infant formula product itself.

Breastfeeding has significant economic consequences at the national level as well as at the family level. It yields savings not only through avoidance of the cost of formula, but also because of averted healthcare costs. A government study estimated that in the U.S., "A minimum of $3.6 billion would be saved if breastfeeding were increased from current levels . . . to those recommended by the U.S. Surgeon General . . . , not counting the savings of the cost of formula. This figure is likely an underestimation of the averted healthcare costs because it represents cost savings from the treatment of only three childhood illnesses ... " (Weimer, 2001, p. 1).

The savings would be even greater if breastfeeding in the U.S. were to follow the recommendations of the World Health Organization. WHO recommends that all infants should be exclusively breastfed for six months, and breastfeeding should be continued, with appropriate complementary feeding, for up to the age of two years or beyond (World Health Organization, 2003). A study in *Pediatrics* estimated that the savings in the U.S. resulting from improved breastfeeding practices would be about $13 billion per year (Bartick & Reinhold, 2010).

Feeding choices have impacts on mothers, families, communities, and others, including corporations. The question then becomes: what benefits for others warrant how much risk to infants over their life spans? The risks and costs of different feeding methods should be weighed on the basis of the best information that can be obtained.

Thus we can identify the first major concern relating to the regulation of infant formula:

ISSUE 1.	Government policy everywhere should recognize that poor health is more likely throughout the lifespan if infants' and young children's diets are based on formula feeding rather than breastfeeding.

3 | The Assumption of Safety

Formula's impacts on children's health depend not only on its composition, but also on how it is distributed, promoted, and used. There is frequent misuse of infant formula as a result of inadequate sanitation, unclean water, and improper mixing. The feeding process itself may not be handled well. The formula manufacturers' position is that they are not responsible if their product is not used as directed. They insist that, apart from exceptional contamination incidents, their product is safe, and if the methods of using it are often unsafe, that is not their responsibility. The regulatory agencies have accepted this claim without serious challenge.

Some people feel that the primary purpose of the Codex Alimentarius Commission and other agencies involved in food regulation really is to facilitate trade in food products by standardizing requirements, with health being a secondary consideration. The industry works to keep the regulations weak, and then claims that their products are safe because they follow the regulations. Blatant violations, such as extreme forms of contamination, are addressed with great fanfare, but many more commonplace issues are ignored.

This is illustrated by the fact that the standards focus on the ingredients in infant formula, but give little attention to the water component. For sterile liquid formula prepared under highly controlled factory conditions, this may not be an important issue. However, most infant formula is prepared at home from powder that is not sterile. Often the water that is used is of questionable quality in high-income, as well as low-income countries. Even if water is of good quality as it arrives in the home, it may be exposed to contamination while in the home. Infant formula that is obtained as a liquid concentrate may or may not be sterile in the container, but it can be contaminated after the container is opened.

There has been concern in the past about contamination from infant formula cans, such as the alarm about lead from the solder once used to seal cans. Now there is growing alarm about plastic containers and feeding bottles because of the bisphenol A in them (IBFAN, 2010; Lunder & Houlihan, 2007). Bisphenol A in infant formula containers has been banned in several jurisdictions (Bardelline, 2011a, 2011b; Keller & Heckman LLP, 2009; Witte, 2011).

Regulators have refused to require warnings on the label that powdered formula is not sterile, and for that reason requires special care in its preparation. Despite the many difficulties that can be encountered in the preparation of infant formula (NCT, 2008; Renfrew, Ansell, & Macleod, 2003), government regulators have done little to require manufacturers to take steps to prevent faulty preparation.

While the international and national regulatory agencies might give the impression that they provide close monitoring to ensure the safety of infant formula, the agencies often simply assume the products are safe. They leave routine testing to the manufacturers.

Even weak monitoring is impractical when infant formula is sold internationally. For example, Wyeth's plant in the U.S. makes no brand name formula for U.S. consumption, but exports the product. Wyeth, now part of Pfizer, Inc., also manufactures infant formula in Ireland for export. Ireland exports a great deal of infant formula and the milk powder used to make infant formula. Ireland exports infant formula to Australia, even while Fonterra's wholly owned branch in Australia also manufactures and exports infant formula. The

Fonterra Co-operative Group is headquartered in New Zealand. It is the world's largest dairy exporter, exporting ingredients for infant formula to Asia and the Middle East. Fonterra manufactures infant formula in many different plants throughout the world.

Ensuring the safety and quality of food products requires traceability–the ability to track products to their source. However, few countries require detailed labeling of the country of origin of the product or of its separate ingredients. Thus, when there are problems with infant formula, it can be difficult to know who to blame or where to go to get the problem fixed.

While the contamination of Chinese infant formula in 2008 is well known, it is not so well known that one of the major Chinese firms involved in the scandal, Sanlu, was 43% owned by Fonterra (Wikipedia, 2011). In 2010 Fonterra was involved in another scandal in China. It supplied milk powder to an infant formula maker whose product was suspected of creating hormonal imbalances in infants (Ramzy, 2010).

The need for oversight of these operations is very clear:

> Financial investigators say there is a long list of small operations – including one running out of a house in Clendon in South Auckland – exporting milk powders and infant formulas....

> New Zealand's vulnerability in China was exposed in 2008 when the partly Fonterra-owned company Sanlu was found to have added melamine to infant formula. Six infants died and 860 needed hospital care.

> One company formed last year, with just 100 shares and whose registered office cannot be found, is sending infant baby formula to China. The baby formula is sold by Kiaora New Zealand International Ltd, under the New Zealand branding of Heitiki (Field, 2011; also see The Economist, 2011).

There are no publicly available data on the patterns of international trade and international investment in infant formula. Without greater transparency, the prospects for monitoring are slim. However, companies that are interested in selling or investing in infant formula can purchase a full package of detailed information from UBIC Consulting for €14,990 (UBIC, 2010).

There is a complicated web of international trade and international investment in infant formula. What rules govern these operations? What quality control is there for infant formula that goes into international trade? The U.S. Food and Drug Administration recognizes the need for a global approach to product safety, but it is much more concerned with the quality of imports into the United States than with the quality of U.S. exports or the responsibilities of the global corporations that the U.S. hosts (U.S. Department of Health and Human Services, 2011f). This is made evident by the fact that under certain conditions infant formula produced in the U.S. for export is exempt from the rules regarding adulteration and misbranding (U.S. Department of Health and Human Services, 2002).

In international relations relating to infant formula, there is a need to monitor not only the actions of manufacturers and investors, but also the actions of governments. Alarming cases have come to light. For example, the U.S.-based Gerber baby food company got the U.S. government to pressure Guatemala's government to weaken its law relating to the *International Code of Marketing of Breast-Milk Substitutes*. It did this by making misleading claims about Guatemala violating international trade agreements (Palmer, 2009, pp. 277-278).

In another case in 2006, when the government of the Philippines was taking legal steps to control the marketing of infant formula,

> [T]he president of the US Chamber of Commerce sent a pressure letter to Pres. Gloria Macapagal Arroyo which implied a possible "risk to reputation of the Philippines as a stable and viable destination for investment."

Health Secretary Francisco T. Duque also shared how officials from the US State Department and the US Embassy approached him and his staff asking for the old provisions to be reinstated so that milk companies can continue business as usual (UNICEF, 2007; also see Monbiot, 2007; Palmer, 2009, pp. 289-292; PCIJ, 2007).

Thus, business interests often trump children's interests, not only within countries, but also in international politics. This pattern is facilitated by the rarely challenged assumption that infant formula is safe to use.

In the U.S., the requirements for many foods, including infant formula, are set out in the Food, Drug, and Cosmetic Act. "All manufacturers of infant formula must begin with safe food ingredients, which are either Generally Recognized As Safe (GRAS) or approved as food additives for use in infant formula" (U.S. Department of Health and Human Services, 2004a).

The concern is only about safety, mainly in the sense of toxicity. Unlike pharmaceuticals, foods do not have to be demonstrated to be effective for their purpose. This issue is taken up later in the chapter on Safety and Nutritional Adequacy. The determination that a product is GRAS means it does not have to be tested for safety before it is marketed.

It is not always the FDA itself that decides. The rule is that "for a food additive, FDA determines the safety of the ingredient; whereas a determination that an ingredient is GRAS can be made by qualified experts outside of government" (U.S. Department of Health and Human Services, 2005, para 4). As the FDA explains,

> The GRAS notification program provides a voluntary mechanism whereby a person may inform FDA of a determination that the use of a substance is GRAS, rather than petition FDA to affirm that the use of a substance is GRAS (U.S. Department of Health and Human Services, 2005, para 8).

Thus, in many cases, the FDA simply takes the word of applicants that the product they wish to have categorized as GRAS should be categorized as safe. There is no assessment by a neutral party. FDA explains its limited role in relation to infant formula as follows:

> FDA does not approve infant formulas before they can be marketed. However, manufacturers of infant formula are subject to FDA's regulatory oversight.
>
> Manufacturers must ensure that infant formula complies with federal nutrient requirements. Manufacturers are required to register with FDA and provide the agency with a notification before marketing a new formula (U.S. Department of Health and Human Services, 2011d, p. 3).

The FDA is not required to do anything with that notification.

Many different foods are routinely accepted as GRAS. Most infant formulas are based on either cow's milk or soymilk, and both of these ingredients are categorized as GRAS. Thus, under this standard, *basic infant formula that includes the required ingredients is assumed to be safe.* The treatment of additives is discussed later in the chapter on Additives.

Dietary safety is based on variety and moderation. The GRAS concept makes some sense when assessing whether a food item is reasonably safe to include in a healthy, diversified adult diet. It is inadequate when that food item *is* the diet. Hamburgers are reasonably safe to eat when they are part of a diverse diet, but as shown in the Morgan Spurlock film, *Super Size Me,* hamburgers are not good for you when they constitute practically the entire diet.

There should be special concern not only because infant formula constitutes practically the entire diet, but also because it is for vulnerable growing infants. Showing that something has been safe for adults does not tell us whether it will be safe for infants.

Soy-based infant formula illustrates the problem. Soymilk has been categorized as GRAS because historically soybeans have been used in the human diet in many forms with no major problems. That categorization was carried over to soy-based infant formula, even though there had been no prior experience with using soymilk as practically the entire diet, whether for adults or for infants.

There have been many problems with soy-based infant formula, but improvements have been made. Several studies assert that it is now safe to use (American Academy of Pediatrics, 2005; Merritt & Jenks, 2004). One report from defenders of soy-based infant formula acknowledges, "some child-advocacy groups claim that consuming soy-based formula could accelerate puberty and cause developmental and reproductive abnormalities and thyroid disorders later in life" (Agricultural Research Service, 2004, p. 8). Their report, "Study Examines Long-Term Health Effects of Soy Infant Formula" describes a six-year study funded by the U.S. Department of Agriculture (Agricultural Research Service, 2004; also see Badger et al., 2009). It is not clear how a six-year study of young children could assess an inherently long-term health effect such as sexual dysfunction. The Agricultural Research Service of the USDA did the study, not a health agency. Agricultural agencies are likely to be more interested than health agencies in promoting the use of soy.

Many reports have raised unanswered questions about the safety of soy, both for the general population (Daniel, 2005) and for infants in particular (British Dietetic Association, 2003; Martyn, 2003; Millington, 2011). The American Academy of Pediatrics has given up its 1998 position in support of soy-based formula and now, with few exceptions, recommends that it should not be used (Bhatia, Greer, & American Academy of Pediatrics Committee on Nutrition, 2008). It is irresponsible for the FDA to simply accept that soy-based infant formula is known to be safe and does not require studies of its safety. Soy is widely accepted as part of the diet for adults, but one should not assume for that reason that it is safe to use as the basis for the entire diet of infants.

While soy has long been used in the human diet, genetically modified soy is new. Nevertheless, it has been categorized as GRAS.

Monsanto has done much of the testing of genetically modified soy (FDA Scientists, 2004). There has been little independent testing.

The use of genetically modified soy in infant formula is even newer than its use in adult diets. Genetically modified soy has been categorized as GRAS, even when it is used as the basic component of infants' entire diet. This assumption certainly does not benefit the infants who consume the formula (Barnett, 2004). Heinz and Wyeth have agreed not to use genetically modified soy in their infant formula (CTV News, 2003; Sarmiento, 2003). In Australia, Greenpeace led a campaign to remove soy-based formula from stores because it was not clearly labeled as using genetically modified ingredients (Lane, 2010).

Major formula companies, such as Nestlé, Mead Johnson, and Ross (Abbott), have used genetically modified ingredients in their infant formula and other infant food products. They defend this practice by saying it meets current safety standards. That does not justify the practice. It raises questions about the adequacy of the standards.

Curiously, in its critique of soy-based formula in 2008, the American Academy of Pediatrics did not discuss the distinctive issues that might arise when it is made from genetically modified soy.

Almost all soy now produced has been genetically modified, so most soy-based infant formula is likely to be based on genetically modified soy, even if that is not acknowledged. This may be why the International Dairy Foods Association no longer says, "because GM ingredients offer no particular benefit over the traditional sources at the present time, IDFA members take all possible steps to ensure that ingredients used in baby foods are not derived from genetically modified crops." The Association no longer says, "Where there is the potential for GM material to be present from, for example, soya or maize, companies source non-GM, identity-preserved ingredients through carefully audited suppliers with independent testing." These statements are no longer on IDFA's website, but at this writing, there were copies at http://www.babymilk.com/children/index.htm and several other websites.

Despite the many questions that have been raised, the FDA has not changed its position. There is a need to challenge the GRAS assumption for soy, and especially for genetically modified soy, in infant formula. Withdrawing the GRAS categorization would not mean soy-based products are unsafe. It would simply acknowledge that the *assumption* of safety is not warranted.

Similarly, no attention has yet been paid to the corn oil and corn syrup solids now common in infant formula. They are almost certainly derived from sources that have been genetically modified. The fungal and algal oils now used to make synthetic DHA and ARA (discussed more fully in the chapter on Additives) are made by genetically modified organisms. The feedstock for cattle producing milk for infant formula is likely to contain ingredients that have been genetically modified.

The FDA generally takes the manufacturers' word that a new food product is safe. It usually does not question the assumption that anything that has been consumed by adults without major problems is safe to add to infant formula.

The uncritical readiness to assume that new variants of infant formula are safe to use is highly questionable and should be challenged. It exposes children to excessive risk.

| **ISSUE 2.** | Safety standards for infant formula should be strengthened. |

4 How Safe Should Formula Be?

Studies consistently show that feeding with infant formula is *less* safe than breastfeeding. That leaves open the question of whether feeding with formula should be regarded as *unsafe*.

Many people assume that in high-income countries, formula feeding is a reasonable second-best choice. That is the position taken by the U.S. Food and Drug Administration (Stehlin, 1996). For many, the choice of second-best is not a big issue. One might argue that the situation is comparable to choosing white rice over brown rice, even though brown rice supposedly is better for you.

There is a major difference, however. For most people, rice is just a part of a diverse diet. There is a good chance that whatever is missing from white rice or any other sub-optimal food will be provided in some other part of the diet. When choosing infant food, however, the choice is made for a food that will constitute the entire diet, or nearly the entire diet, of the infant for six months or more during a critical formative period. Infant formula is often also used as a major nutrient source well after children start taking other foods. The risks of making a wrong choice are much higher when the diet is not diverse. White rice is safe to eat, but a diet of white rice alone is not.

In terms of its impact on child health, breastfeeding is best. Optimal breastfeeding means early initiation (in the first hour after birth), exclusive breastfeeding for six months, and continued breastfeeding for up to two years or more (World Health Organization, 2003). The Infant Formula Council, a formula industry group based in the U.S., says, "if a mother cannot or chooses not to exclusively breastfeed for six months—an iron-fortified infant formula is the only safe alternative" (Infant Formula Council, 2010). That is not correct. In terms of the infant's health, second best is expressed breast-milk from the biological mother. Third best is wet-nursing, meaning breastfeeding by a woman who is not the biological mother. Infant formula comes in fourth. Of course, in terms of infants with special needs or considerations other than the child's health, such as the mother's convenience or her need to go to work, formula might be ranked higher.

There is a newly emerging option that probably should be in fourth place, bumping infant formula to fifth place. This is the provision of breast-milk from mother to mother (Akre, Gribble, & Minchin, 2011). Craig's List and other marketing devices are now being used to promote sales of frozen breast-milk. There is now a website facilitating this trade, at http://www.onlythebreast.com/.

The choices among alternative feeding methods are crucially important in addressing the serious malnutrition among young children in many parts of the world. In some low-income countries, where food security is a serious problem, some young children are being provided with Ready to Use Therapeutic Foods, such as Plumpy'Nut. There is serious concern that such foods might displace breastfeeding and traditional local foods (BDNews, 2011; Latham, Jonsson, Sterken, & Kent, 2011). If it were not for the commercial interests behind such products, perhaps more effort would be devoted to promoting continued breastfeeding. The displacement of breastfeeding is one of the major concerns driving recent efforts to formulate guidelines for both Ready to Use Therapeutic Foods (RUTFs) and Ready to Use Supplementary Foods (RUSFs) (Emergency Nutrition Network, 2011).

To ensure the availability of breast-milk beyond six months, it is important to promote exclusive breastfeeding for the first six months. Niger, one of the hungriest nations in the world, would not have so many malnourished young children if it had a higher rate of exclusive breastfeeding of infants (Kristof, 2011), and more continued breastfeeding beyond six months.

When Médecins Sans Frontières promoted the use of Plumpy'Nut to treat malnourished children in Niger, they based their argument on the fact that it was better for children than the corn-soy mix that was provided through food aid programs (Isanaka et al., 2009; Latham, 2011; Médecins Sans Frontières, 2008). However, they did not compare Plumpy'Nut with better breastfeeding practices and better use of local foods. This is similar to the device of boasting about a new version of infant formula by comparing it with an older version, and avoiding any comparison with breastfeeding.

Commercial ready-to-use foods may be promoted for use in emergency situations with a view to creating demand for the products when the emergency has passed. This concern is illustrated by the World Food Programme's promotion of Plumpy'Doz:

> WFP delivered Plumpy'Doz to children in Ouagadougou and Bobo Dioulasso through an innovative voucher system. In 2009, 360 metric tons of the ready-to-use, nutritious food supplement were distributed to more than 40,000 children under two –20,237 girls and 20,089 boys. Health centres in these locations report better nutrition among children who have received the specialised product, a paste supplement made from vegetable fat, peanut butter, sugar, and milk. Burkinabe children, who have grown fond of the supplement, have nicknamed it "chocolate" (World Food Programme, 2010, p. 28).

These vouchers might be a way of distributing free samples in anticipation of marketing these products as a new kind of treat.

Similar nutritional benefits might have been obtained with better breastfeeding and better use of local foods.

There are concerns, for high-income as well as low-income countries, about the displacement of breastfeeding due to the use of formula, toddler milks, yogurts, and other manufactured foods for children beyond six months of age. Breastfeeding is important for these young children, just as it is for infants under six months. As Pamela Morrison points out, breastfeeding beyond six months "still provides the most important source of good-quality protein, vitamins A and C, calcium, and the long chain polyunsaturated fatty acids that are unobtainable from any other source (Morrison, 2001, p. 30; also see Williams, 2005).

There seems to be a pattern of avoiding comparisons with breastfeeding. In the U.S., the Institute of Medicine argues that infant formula, "although inferior to human milk in multiple respects, promotes more efficient growth, development, and nutrient balance than commercially available cow milk" (Institute of Medicine, 2004, p. 42). While this is certainly true, it is not a compelling argument for using infant formula. Just as attention should be given to the differences in impacts on child health and development between feeding with infant formula and feeding with cow milk, attention should be given to the differences between feeding with infant formula and feeding with breast-milk.

In high-income countries, such as the U.S., many parents' experience tells them that using formula is safe. Neighbors feed their infants' formula, and they seem to do well. People tend to assume that if the government allows the product to be sold, it must be safe.

Risk management by governments can be based on scientific evidence and analysis, but individuals tend to operate on a more intuitive basis. The general public's concerns regarding food safety tend to focus on specific contaminants that lead to identifiable adverse events. These events often have intense and immediate consequences in terms of illness and death. They sometimes affect relatively few people. Often it is possible to locate the bad food, and then trace a direct causal connection between the food and the adverse health consequences.

There have been many cases of dangerous contamination of infant formula. In recent years, a number of *Enterobacter sakazakii* infections and deaths among infants were traced to contaminated milk-based powdered infant formulas. People always become alarmed when they learn that defective infant formula has been distributed, whether because of manufacturing errors or outright fraud, as in the case of the melamine-laced Chinese infant formula in 2008.

Risks are difficult to communicate (Esterik, 2002; Leiss & Powell, 2004), so stories about long-term nutritional inadequacy (discussed later in the chapter on Safety and Nutritional Adequacy) get little attention. The Institute of Medicine has formulated detailed guidelines for evaluating the *safety* of new ingredients added to infant formula (Institute of Medicine, 2004), but it has offered no guidelines for assessing the *nutritional adequacy or effectiveness* of additives or any specific type of infant formula.

We should be pleased that agencies, such as the U.S. Food and Drug Administration, track food-related illnesses and deaths, such as those associated with identifiable pathogens. They should give similar attention to the illnesses and deaths associated with dietary patterns. Many governments are now tracking the causes and consequences of overweight, but the impacts of infant feeding choices are not getting nearly as much attention. Perhaps this is because the economic forces at work do not stand to gain from optimizing infants' diets.

The cumulative effect of dietary choices can add up to much greater total harm than the dramatic short-term high impact events, such as contamination, but the harms are more difficult to detect. To draw an analogy, worldwide, there is far more human misery attributable to the lack of clean water than to terrorism, but terrorism gets far more play in the news. More systematic research should be done to assess long-term impacts of different diets for infants and young children.

For some people, the impact of long-term risks can be grasped more readily when they are described in terms of costs. Several studies have compared the likely costs of healthcare with different methods of child feeding (Bartick & Reinhold, 2010; Weimer, 2001).

Is the fact that formula feeding leads to more infant deaths and illnesses than breastfeeding something to be alarmed about, or should we take it in stride, the way we accept automobile accident fatalities, for example? Individuals can make their own judgments, of course, but how can one make a more scientific analysis?

In examining the safety of formula feeding when compared with breastfeeding, the first task is to be clear about what kind of risks there are. The Agency for Healthcare Research and Quality, for example, reported that in the U.S., formula feeding leads to increased risks of necrotizing enterocolitis, otitis media, gastroenteritis, hospitalization for lower respiratory tract infections, atopic dermatitis, sudden infant death syndrome, childhood asthma, childhood leukemia, type 1 diabetes mellitus, and childhood obesity (Bartick & Reinhold, 2010).

Others take a more global view, adding other concerns (INFACT Canada, 2002). The list could be extended further if long-term health and developmental outcomes were considered. One could also refine the list by talking about variations in the types and degrees of these possible outcomes. Apart from the health-related outcomes themselves, one could also talk about the risks of incurring high healthcare costs.

The different *types* of risk associated with using infant formula should be matters of concern everywhere. The actual *degree* of risk associated with each type varies under different circumstances, and can be estimated only with high quality research in defined populations. The risks generally are lower in high-income places than they are in low-income places. They vary with different kinds of living circumstances and may depend on genetic factors, so different ethnic groups may have different levels of risk for that reason alone.

Apart from genetic factors, there is a great deal of variation among ethnic groups in their breastfeeding practices and in their living circumstances. For example, in the U.S., African-Americans breastfeed at a much lower rate than whites. This, together with their tendency to have low birth-weight infants, helps to explain why African-Americans have much higher child mortality rates.

Earlier we said that in terms of the infant's health, breastfeeding is best, second best is expressed breast-milk from the biological mother, third best is wet-nursing, and infant formula comes in fourth or maybe fifth. The problem with this sort of ranking is that it conveys no sense of the distance between the alternatives. The simple ranking may be misleading if one assumes that they are bunched closely together, with only small differences among them.

Careful research is needed to assess the degree of difference in risks between different feeding methods. Those differences are likely to vary in different contexts. However, on the basis of the scientific information that has been accumulated so far, it seems reasonable to estimate that all the options based on breast-milk are close to one another, and, in comparison, infant formula is considerably worse in terms of its likely impact on infants' health.

There are several different ways to describe the risk of choosing one feeding method when compared with another. For example, in the U.S. Surgeon General's *Call to Action to Support Breastfeeding*, an appendix on Excess Health Risks Associated with Not Breastfeeding describes Excess Risk as a percentage (U.S. Department of Health and Human Services, 2011b, p. 79). Thus, the table says that children who have *never* been breastfed are 32 percent more likely to be obese than children who have *ever* been breastfeed. Figures of that sort are provided for a number of other outcomes of concern.

McNiel, Labbok, and Abraham's study (2010) of the risks associated with formula feeding when compared with exclusive breastfeeding illustrates another way of talking about degrees of risk. Their review of available U.S.-based studies allowed them to estimate *odds ratios* to describe the relative risks associated with using formula. For example, according to their sources, the odds ratio for otitis media in the first six months was 4.55. This means that, in the population studied, infants who were fed any amount of formula were 4.55 times as likely to have otitis media as exclusively breastfed infants. Odds ratios were also estimated for diabetes, asthma, and other health issues.

When talking about the relative risks for various health outcomes with different methods of infant feeding, it is important to be clear about what is being compared. The odds ratio for otitis media would be different if feeding with a particular type of infant formula was being compared with exclusive breastfeeding, feeding with another type of infant formula, or feeding with cow's milk.

Just as there are different types of infant formula and different ways of using them, there are distinctions to be made among ways of breastfeeding. In some studies, the comparison is to infants who have ever breastfed, as in the *Surgeon General's Call to Action to Support Breastfeeding* (U.S. Department of Health and Human Services, 2011b, p. 79). In other studies (e.g., McNiel, Labbok, & Abrahams, 2010), the comparison is to infants who have been exclusively breastfed for a specific number of months. People often speak simply about comparing formula feeding and breastfeeding, but to really compare the risks, it is important to specify the character of both in some detail.

The infant formula manufacturers directly or indirectly sponsor much of the research on infant formula. It is almost always limited to comparing one class of formula with another. Few studies compare the health impacts of infant formula with that of exclusive or predominant breastfeeding. Few studies look at long-term impacts. It is important to recognize that when formula manufacturers make claims about the "benefits" provided by their products, they are always talking about comparisons with other types of formula. Apart from their cursory initial acknowledgment that breast is best, they never seriously compare formula feeding with breastfeeding. They do not provide the information that is needed to help guide the choice between formula feeding and breastfeeding.

It is not only the manufacturers that are at fault. Few government agencies do anything to provide women with quality information to help guide the choice. They avoid dealing with the question by framing their discussions in terms of what women should do if they cannot or choose not to breastfeed.

Risk estimates are averages based on the historical record for a specific population. They do not say what the risks are for any individual child. Also, they do not hold if the living conditions of that population change significantly. For example, the risks of using infant formula in China as it becomes wealthier should not be estimated on the basis of data collected when it was much poorer.

The risks are not distributed evenly within the population. The poor and some other groups generally face higher than average risks, while high-income people tend to face lower risks.

It is useful to obtain numerical estimates of the risks and benefits of taking one course of action when compared with another course of action. However, there may be some risks and benefits that are not easily quantified. Numerical data should be used carefully. The assessment of the numbers should be accompanied by carefully considered judgments that take into account other factors that might not have been captured by the data.

Most people are not used to thinking about risk in a systematic way. As individuals, we are not in a position to collect the data needed to estimate risks. This is the task of government. No other agency is in a position to collect systematic, fair, objective data on a large scale in a sustained way. Even then, there may be reason for doubts. Often private interests have a way of influencing governments' efforts to assemble and analyze data, or preventing that collection altogether.

Having good data available on the risks associated with not breastfeeding is important, but it is not enough. There is also a need to have some systematic way of making the judgment, based on the data, as to whether using formula is acceptable or not. The question could be asked about a particular type of infant formula or about the use of infant formula in general. One study estimated that in the U.S. there are about 911 excess infant deaths each year that could be averted with proper breastfeeding (Bartick & Reinhold, 2010). Is that a trivial number or a cause for alarm? How should that judgment be made?

There is a need for guidance for individual decision-making and also for making public policy. For example, in the United States, section 412(e) of the Federal Food, Drug, and Cosmetic (21 U.S.C. 350a(e)) provides that if the Secretary of Health and Human Services determines that the infant formula presents a risk to human health, the manufacturer must immediately recall that infant formula. How much risk? What kinds of risks? There is no guidance on what type and level of risk should be regarded as significant enough to warrant the recall of the product. The regulations say that "when an adulterated or misbranded infant formula presents a risk to human health, a manufacturer shall immediately take all actions necessary to recall that formula" (Burrows, 2007, p. 6), but there is no guidance on other types of risks or how to assess the degree of risk.

Perhaps the FDA is not greatly concerned about weighing the risks to infants' health. As of the middle of 2011 its records showed that there were only five manufacturers of infant formula in the U.S., and on average, there were only two infant formula recalls per year in the preceding three years (U.S. Federal Register, 2011).

Other agencies could have been more helpful in addressing the question of when infant formula should be regarded as unsafe. To illustrate, when the Academy of Breastfeeding Medicine set out detailed "Educational Objectives and Skills for the Physician with Respect to Breastfeeding" (Academy of Breastfeeding Medicine, 2011), its detailed guidance did not say anything about how physicians might compare alternative methods of feeding or how they might support pregnant women in making informed choices of feeding methods. It would have been helpful if the Academy addressed the broader issue of infant feeding, not just breastfeeding.

In relation to infant feeding, one expert said, "The whole notion of talking about risk is new in this field, but it's the only field of public health, except perhaps physical activity, where there is never any talk about the risk" (Rabin, 2006). One can only speculate on why that is so. Why haven't health professionals and agencies of government encouraged more systematic comparisons of the impacts of formula feeding and breastfeeding, in the long-term as well as the short term?

It would make sense to compare governments' risk management of infant formula with that provided for other products. When even a small number of deaths is associated with defective toys or contaminated foods, those products are recalled very quickly. Should infant formula be treated differently? Why is it that the U.S. Consumer Product Safety Commission recalled and then banned drop-side cribs because they caused 32 infant deaths over a ten-year period (Martin, 2011; Johnson, 2011), but U.S. government agencies seem unconcerned by the estimated 911 feeding-related deaths of children each year? If infant formula were to be categorized as a pharmaceutical or a dietary supplement, would the FDA withdraw it from the market?

We don't have a clear consensus on when particular practices should be judged to be unsafe and thus in need of some sort of public policy intervention. There is room for debate about what should be considered a troubling risk. One way to handle this might be to agree that if children fed with infant formula show a *statistically significant* higher level of morbidity or mortality than breastfed infants in the same population, this is an indicator of *significant* risk. In such cases, the choice of feeding methods should become a matter of public policy concern. If using infant formula entails measurable and systematic risk for the health of children, restrictions on its distribution should be considered.

The public policy interventions could range from warnings to total prohibition of use of the product, with many possible variations in between. Its availability could be restricted, so that it is sold only in pharmacies, and perhaps only by prescription, as is the case in some countries. In many countries, special infant formulas for infants with unique needs are available only by prescription. Some people feel all infant formula should be made available only by prescription (Miles & Betts, 2010). Others feel that any restrictions would constitute an excessive intrusion into the freedom of choice and interfere with free trade.

It would be sensible to agree that *governments should take responsibility for protecting their people from extreme risks, but people should be free to choose when the risks are small.* Thus, governments should protect us from dangerously contaminated rice, but leave us free to choose between white rice and brown rice.

For risks that are short of the extreme levels that might trigger governmental recall of products, governments should ensure that people obtain good information that would help them make their own informed choices.

Choices among different feeding methods should be informed choices, regardless of whether the decision-makers are parents or government officials. Governments have a responsibility to ensure that the best possible information is made available.

Governments should provide clear and fair information that would help individuals and government agencies compare the impacts of formula feeding and breastfeeding. Governments should also provide information that would help people and agencies deal with significant differences among different infant formulas. So far, neither the general public nor the regulatory agencies have been provided with information of the quality and the form they would need to make good informed choices.

When formula feeding and breastfeeding are presented as if they are nearly equal choices, parents and regulatory agencies are misled. Using formula involves real risks, and the risks should be taken seriously. Parents may reasonably choose to expose their infants to small risks in exchange for other kinds of benefits, just as they take risks each time they take their infants into their cars. If we pretend that there are no risks, we mislead parents into exposing their infants to far greater risks than they would if they were well informed.

Parents should be assumed to be competent decision-makers. They should be supported in making informed choices with good information and sensible suggestions about how to handle that information. They should never be exposed to misleading information, especially information that is deliberately misleading. There is a need for entirely new methods of regulation, based on the precautionary principle, meaning that where there is uncertainty, policies should favor the children. Where there is a choice to be made, manufacturers should bear the risks, not the children.

Many people have said that artificial feeding is the largest uncontrolled *in vivo* experiment in human history. However, in scientific experiments, the relevant data are systematically collected and analyzed. This has never been done. Systematic monitoring of the actual performance, over time, of specific infant formulas in comparison with breastfeeding seems to have been deliberately avoided, despite the huge amounts of resources allocated to food-related research throughout the world. As pointed out later in the chapter on Additives, even when the United States' Food and Drug Administration tells manufacturers "to monitor, through scientific studies and rigorous post-market surveillance," the manufacturers fail to do that, and the agency does not challenge them about that failure.

Maureen Minchin speculates that if thorough and fair research was undertaken, "everyone will agree that the risks of formula are unacceptable except where truly avoidable" (Minchin, 1998a, p. 31).

James Akre has a similar view:

> Running the numbers successfully and interpreting their significance accurately should serve as a tipping point–for achieving the critical mass required to reverse trends towards artificial feeding in some environments; for increasing breastfeeding prevalence and duration in others; and for restructuring the healthcare system, community, and workplace in ways to ensure that, because these changes are understood to be in the best interest of society as a whole, they are welcomed by one and all. International public health nutrition policy

needs to promote cost-effective decision making by ensuring that the science-based understanding of the health – and therefore the economic – implications of more or less breastfeeding are thoroughly assessed, convincingly presented, and taken fully into account (Akre 2006, 2009, p. 14).

The McNiel, Labbok, and Abraham (2010) data on risks associated with formula feeding were pieced together from available published reports. It would be much easier to obtain meaningful odds ratio information if new data were to be collected specifically for that purpose. Data could be collected not only for countries, but also for smaller sub-national populations, such as states or even communities.

If government agencies were motivated to compare the risks of different feeding methods, the data could be assembled through systems already in place. They could coordinate data collections through health service agencies. The U.S. has a well-developed Pediatric Nutrition Surveillance System specifically designed to "monitor the nutritional status of low-income infants, children, and women in federally funded maternal and child health programs" (PEDNSS, 2011, para 1). With modifications, it could be used to compare short-term and long-term health outcomes with different methods of feeding.

The Millennium Cohort Study in the UK already collects data on infant feeding that can be related to a broad variety of other variables they collect, such as child behavior, cognitive development, and child and parental health (Millennium, 2011). To illustrate, a study based on that data collection examined relationships between child feeding methods and child behavior (Heikkilä, Sacker, Kelly, Renfrew, & Quigley, 2011). That collection could be used to systematically estimate a number of risks associated with different methods of infant feeding.

Large health maintenance organizations could assemble the data that are needed quite easily. Similarly, the United States' Special

Supplemental Nutrition Program for Women, Infants, and Children could organize data collections so that comparisons could be made of the health status of children that have been fed in different ways. Doing that would help the program to carry out its health-centered mission.

ISSUE 3.	Public policy should limit the exposure of children to excessive risk. Mothers should receive guidance to help them take risk considerations into account when deciding how to feed their children.

5 Outdated and Counterfeit Infant Formula

Even if a product is of good quality when it is manufactured, it may not stay that way. Powdered infant formula is not a sterile product, and it deteriorates over time. Therefore, the Codex standards for infant formula specify in paragraph 9.4.1:

> The date of minimum durability (preceded by the words "best before") shall be declared by the day, month, and year in uncoded numerical sequence except that for products with a shelf-life of more than three months, the month and year will suffice (Codex Alimentarius Commission, 2007).

Similarly, regulations under the U.S. Federal Food, Drug, and Cosmetic Act require that a "use by" or expiration date must be indicated on each container of infant formula. FDA recommends that infant formula past the "use by" date should not be sold. There is nothing in U.S. national law that prohibits the sale of outdated infant formula.

The high price of infant formula has prompted many deliberate contamination cases, thefts (Schneider, 2010), and other abuses of the product.

In some cases, the criminality goes to extremes:

> Unethical marketing practices sometimes take criminal dimension when low quality or expired breast-milk substitutes are sold, putting children in double jeopardy. In 2001, a world-renowned manufacturer of infant formula imported in Nigeria nine 40-feet containers of expired skimmed milk powder to be used in the production of breast-milk substitutes. Without the vigilance of the National Agency for Food and Drug Administration and Control (NAFDAC), the expired milk would have been used and sold to the unsuspecting public. Another case was that of a man in Abuja who was mixing cassava flour, milk, and sugar, and packing it in recycled containers of breast-milk substitutes. He confessed that he had done that for years (Sokol, Aquayo, & Clark, 2007, p. v).

In 1995 in the U.S.:

> A SEVEN-MONTH Government investigation has uncovered extensive scams to market bogus, outdated, or mislabeled baby formula, and there are indications that other counterfeit products, from shampoo to coffee to prescription drugs, are also being sold to unsuspecting consumers.
>
> The baby-formula investigation, begun by the Food and Drug Administration after 45,000 pounds of counterfeit infant formula was seized in California in February, has uncovered at least 10 operations in eight states that have apparently sold bogus formula by having it made by small producers and placed in cans with counterfeit labels (Burros, 1995).

National governments have acted in some high-profile cases, such as the melamine contamination of infant formula in China, but on the whole, national governments and international agencies do not do enough to control such behaviors. The weak response is well illustrated by the U.S. Food and Drug Administration. In 2009 it issued a Notice to Retailers regarding the sale of outdated infant formula, saying, "Such formula should be pulled off of the retail shelf" (U.S. Department of Health and Human Services, 2009, para 2). It could not say such sales were illegal under federal law because it is not illegal. The exact same letter had been circulated ten years earlier.

In most states of the United States, there is no law against selling outdated infant formula (Di Mesio, 2008; Young, 1998; Young, 2000). In California and New York, Attorneys General found a number of stores selling outdated infant formula and other baby foods (State of California, 2008). In 2009 the Consumer Federation of California sponsored a bill that would have prohibited such sales, but Governor Schwarzenegger vetoed the bill. In New Jersey, however, "Wal-Mart, following a finding that it sold or offered to sell expired baby formula and non-prescription drugs to consumers, has entered into settlement with the state to pay $775,000 and revise its business practices to comply with state laws and regulations" (Hester, 2010, para 1).

The requirement for placing a "best before" or "use by" date on infant formula might lead some people to believe that there is a control system in place. However, in most places, there are no regulations to prevent misuse of outdated or defective infant formula. There are few laws against selling outdated formula. There are no specifications as to what must be done with outdated or recalled formula. There is no systematic tracking of the disposition of outdated or recalled infant formula.

Some of the infant formula sold in low-income countries might have been shipped there after becoming outdated in high-income countries. In some shops, one can find cartons of infant formula with small stickers strategically placed over the printed use-by date.

The ambiguity of the rules regarding outdated infant formula in most places may be contrasted with Botswana's Food Control Act, which says, in Part II, paragraph 7 of its *Marketing of Foods for*

Infants and Young Children Regulations, 2005, "No person shall stock, distribute, sell or exhibit any foods for infants and young children which have expired or are beyond their shelf life."

A strong system of regulation could limit sale or other distribution of outdated and counterfeit infant formula, and also prescribe methods of disposition of such products. Measures could be taken to improve the traceability of infant formula. Regulations could establish requirements for careful record keeping of the chain of custody until the product is disposed of under prescribed rules. Some alternative uses of the product might be allowed, such as using it in animal feed.

ISSUE 4.   Stronger measures should be taken to limit the use of outdated and counterfeit infant formula.

Nourishing and Nurturing

Infant formula is not as good for infants as breast-milk. However, the comparison really should be between formula *feeding* and breast *feeding*, since the benefits of the breastfeeding process go beyond those delivered by the fluid itself.

A conceptual framework for explaining child malnutrition is provided in Figure 6.1:

> The major underlying causes of child malnutrition, portrayed in the horizontal line of three ovals, are related to *food, care* practices, and *health* services. Focusing exclusively on the chemical composition of breast-milk or infant formula would mean focusing on the food and neglecting the other two key factors contributing to good nutrition. For infants and young children, the care component, or what we call nurturance, is particularly important. Attention should be given to nurturance as well as to the nutrition provided by food (Engle, Menon, & Haddad, 1997).

It is not just *what* is fed, but also *how* that matters. In infant feeding, close body contact is

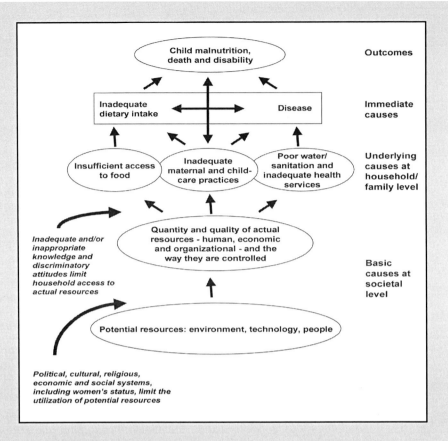

Figure 6.1. Causes of Child Malnutrition

Source: United Nations Children's Fund. (1998). *The state of the world's children,* as reproduced in Pelletier, David L. (2002). *Toward a common understanding of malnutrition: Assessing the contributions of the UNICEF framework.* New York and Washington, D.C.: UNICEF and World Bank. http://www.tulane.edu/~internut/publications/WB_Bckgrd_Pprs/Narrative/NarrativeonePelletierfinal.doc Also available in World Food Programme 2000. *Food and nutrition handbook.* Rome, Italy: WFP, 23-25. http://foodquality.wfp.org/FoodNutritionalQuality/WFPNutritionPolicy/tabid/362/Default.aspx?PageContentID=537

especially important. While contact is possible when feeding formula with a bottle, often children are simply given a bottle, and the mother attends to other matters, perhaps with the child sucking on a bottle propped on a pillow. This can happen with formula in the bottle or expressed breast-milk in the bottle. However, this cannot happen with direct breastfeeding. In general, the quality of care is likely to be lower with formula feeding (Kennell & Klaus, 1998; Smith & Ellwood, 2009; Thorley, 2011).

In some contexts, there may be a need to go beyond providing advice and to establish clear rules for hospitals, clinics, and other facilities to protect and facilitate nurturance. Women who have children in hospitals, prisons, or any other settings should be enabled not only to feed their children, but also to nurture them (Women's Prison Association, 2009). When we see that in some cases new mothers have to pay a bribe to be with their infants, it becomes clear that strong measures may be needed to protect women's right to be with their infants (Dugger, 2005). Several elements of the Baby Friendly Hospital Initiative address the need to facilitate the nurturance, and not only the nutrition of infants (Baby Friendly USA, 2011; UNICEF, 2011).

ISSUE 5.	Mothers should be advised regarding methods of feeding that are nurturing for the children. Where it is appropriate, rules should be established to ensure that agencies enable the nurturing relationship.

7 Additives

Focusing on standard infant formula's lack of fatty acids, manufacturers now add synthetic docosahexaenoic acid and arachidonic acid, commonly known as DHA and ARA. The primary manufacturer is Martek Biosciences Corporation, part of DSM Nutritional Products:

> Naturally present in human breast-milk, DHA (docosahexaenoic acid), and ARA (arachidonic acid) are fatty acids important to infant development and growth. Clinical studies have demonstrated numerous benefits for infants receiving DHA and ARA supplemented formula, including improved mental and visual development. Martek's blend of DHA and ARA, life'sDHA & life'sARA, is the only source of these nutrients currently used in U.S. infant formula, and is present in more than 95 percent of infant formula sold in the U.S. Additionally, Martek is a leading global supplier of DHA and ARA and infant formulas containing Martek's nutritional oils are available in more than 75 countries worldwide (Martek, 2009a, para 4; also see Martek, 2011).

Martek's versions of DHA and ARA are now used in many different food products, for adults as well as for children.

Martek says DHA and ARA are important in infant development, which is certainly correct, but that is knowledge about the natural form of these fatty acids, as they occur in breast-milk. Synthetic forms that are used as food additives might not be effective. Serious doubts have been raised about Martek's claim that, "Clinical studies have demonstrated numerous benefits for infants receiving DHA and ARA supplemented formula, including improved mental and visual development" (Martek, 2009a, para 4; 2009b, para 3; 2009c, para 5). Benefits compared to what? The promotional material is ambiguous, possibly leading some people to believe that these additives make infant formula equal to or maybe even better than breast-milk.

Some studies suggest benefits from the addition of such long-chain polyunsaturated fatty acids to infant formula when compared to infant formula without that additive (Willatts, Forsyth, Di Modugno, Varma, & Colvin, 1998). Other studies show no effect (Lucas et al., 1999). Many experts say the addition of synthetic DHA/ARA to infant formula has not been demonstrated to produce benefits either for pre-term infants or full-term infants (Simmer, Schulzke, & Patole, 2008; Simmer, Patole, & Rao, 2008). Moreover, there are reasons for caution about adding them to infant formula, including possible harm to infants' health and unnecessary increases in cost (Heinig, Goldbronn, & Bañuelos, 2010; Vallaeys, 2008, 2010).

The Institute of Medicine was able to foresee that the supporters of additives might try to compare formulas with new additives only with older formulas, and not with breastfeeding:

> The committee anticipates that manufacturers will wish to add both ingredients that are currently contained in human milk, but not in formulas (e.g., LC-PUFAs), and those not found in human milk (e.g., prebiotics) to enhance the performance of formulas to a level at or nearer to human milk. Thus a breastfed control group should be part of experimental designs

to assess the addition of ingredients new to infant formulas in order to provide a performance standard.

From a regulatory standpoint, the effect of an ingredient new to infant formulas is usually driven by a manufacturer's desire to produce products that mimic the advantages of breastfeeding. This motivation implies that formula in its current state is inferior (e.g., relatively neurologically or immunologically less beneficial, although not necessarily unsafe) when compared with human milk. Thus the safety (and efficacy) of any addition of an ingredient new to infant formulas will need to be judged against two control groups: one fed the previous iteration of the formula without the added ingredient, and one breastfed (Institute of Medicine, 2004, p. 51).

This advice has not been heeded. The manufacturers do not make scientific comparisons of feeding with any of their products with breastfeeding. The FDA and other regulatory agencies do not require the manufacturers or any other organization to make such comparisons. While randomized controlled trials might be ethically questionable, it would be possible to undertake careful observational studies to assess the merits of different methods of feeding.

The doubts about the claims regarding DHA and ARA have led to legal challenges, including a challenge to Mead Johnson for claiming, "only Enfamil LIPIL is clinically proven to improve brain and eye development" (Zale, 2011, para 4). How could it be that only their brand is effective? How would they know that? What published independent scientific studies support such a claim?

Maureen Minchin observes, "Each new version of these fatty acids, produced by different organisms and extracted by patented processes to make different formulations, will be different from the previous one, and the results of studies for one cannot be assumed to apply to any other. Martek needed to reformulate their product after it caused adverse reactions, including intractable diarrhoea, when used in so-called hypo-allergenic formula, for example" (M. Minchin, personal communication, 2011).

Similar issues arise with other additives (or "supplements") to infant formula, such as prebiotics and probiotics (Collier, 2009; Probiotic, 2011; Shafai, 2009). Many additives have unproven benefits and expose infants to new kinds of risks. Many appear to be designed to exploit parents' willingness to pay higher prices to gain every real or imagined benefit for their children.

There are endless claims to improvements to particular types of infant formula, but little acknowledgment that the previous versions might have been deficient. One study even suggested that, "addition of human milk proteins to infant formula may be necessary to obtain some of the nutritional and health benefits that breastfed infants enjoy" (Lönnerdal, 2002, p. 218S). It then proposed genetic modification of plants to produce recombinant human milk proteins that could then be added to infant formula.

In another effort to perfect breast-milk substitutes, "Chinese scientists announced the development of genetically modified dairy cows capable of producing milk with the characteristics of human milk" (Earthweek, 2011, para 1; also see Good Food, 2011). These attempts to create "humanized milk" go back several decades. The studies do not discuss the idea that it might be easier, cheaper, and better for infants to be breastfed.

In dealing with additives and other variations in infant formula, it is important to distinguish what changes or additions to the *composition* of infant formula are allowed from the question of what *claims* are allowed.

In the U.S. Nutrition Labeling and Education Act of 1990, which amended the Food, Drug, and Cosmetic Act, a distinction is made between nutrient content claims and health claims. Nutrient content claims characterize the level of a nutrient in a food. Health claims characterize a relationship of a nutrient to a disease or health-related condition.

U.S. rules regarding health claims have been summarized as follows:

> The U.S. Food and Drug Administration's regulatory authority over health claims was clarified in 1990 legislation known as the Nutrition Labeling and Education Act (NLEA). This law established mandatory nutrition labeling for most foods and placed restrictions on the use of food label claims characterizing the levels or health benefits of nutrients in foods. NLEA set a high threshold for the scientific standard under which the U.S. Food and Drug Administration (FDA) may authorize health claims, this standard is known as the significant scientific agreement (SSA) standard. Subsequent legislation known as the Food and Drug Administration Modernization Act (FDAMA) provided an alternative to FDA review of the health claim where an U.S. government scientific body other than FDA concluded that there is SSA for a substance/disease relationship. Courts have since extended the scope of health claims to include qualified health claims (QHC) that are health claims not substantiated on evidence that meets the level of SSA standard, but include a qualifying statement intended to convey to the consumer the level of evidence for the claim. FDA has responded by developing an evidence-based ranking system for scientific data to determine the level of evidence substantiating a health claim (Rowlands & Hoadley, 2006, p. 1).

Comparable regulations of health claims came into force for the European Union in January 2007 (Reuterswärd, 2007).

Claims must be restricted to prevent manufacturers from making claims that are not well supported scientifically. Often new claims are associated with increased prices that may be unjustified. Because of these concerns, under European Union rules, such claims are supposed to be restricted in accordance with the *International Code of Marketing of Breast-Milk Substitutes* (EUR-Lex, 2011).

Attention should be given to the legality of claims about all foods intended for children. To illustrate, a warning letter from the U.S. Food and Drug Administration to the Beech-Nut Nutrition Corporation listed some of the company's products, and said:

> We have concluded that these products are in violation of the Federal Food, Drug, and Cosmetic Act (the Act) and FDA regulations. . . . Specifically, the above-listed products are misbranded within the meaning of section 403(r)(1)(A) of the Act [21 USC 343(r)(1)(A)] because their labeling includes unauthorized nutrient content claims. Except for claims regarding percentages of vitamins and minerals for which there is an established Reference Daily Intake, a nutrient content claim cannot be made for a food that is intended for use by infants and children less than two years of age unless the claim is specifically provided for in parts 101, 105, or 107 of the regulations. 21 CFR 101.13(b)(3). . . .

> The circumstances under which these claims are permitted are defined in 21 CFR 101.60(c) and 101.54(e), respectively. However, those regulations do not permit these claims for products intended for infants and children under age 2 (U.S. Department of Health and Human Services, 2010c).

While this warning letter to Beech-Nut did not speak directly about infant formula, it raises questions about the legal status of manufacturers' claims about synthetic DHA/ARA and other supplements to infant formula. Following the practice in a number of other countries, in 2001 the U.S. Food and Drug Administration accepted the addition of DHA to infant formulas. However, it has not affirmed that this addition is beneficial, and it has not authorized the manufacturers to make claims regarding their benefits. Some of the current claims might violate the law cited in the FDA's letter to

Beech-Nut, located in the U.S. Code of Federal Regulations at 21 CFR 101.13(b)(3).

Questions about the claims regarding DHA and ARA's role in improving visual acuity have been raised in the European Union. The European Food Safety Authority (EFSA) examined several claims in its *Scientific Opinions on DHA and ARA and Visual Development, Lipil and Visual Development, and Enfamil Premium and Visual Development.* In each case, EFSA supported the same claim regarding the scientific evidence: "DHA contributes to the visual development of infants" (EFSA Panel on Dietetic Products, Nutrition and Allergies, 2009, para 14).

The European Parliament's Committee on Environment, Public Health and Food Safety objected to EFSA's finding saying,

> . . . there is no proven link between artificially added DHA and eyesight, and some studies have found possible negative effects of DHA supplementation.

> As the scientific evidence is still inconclusive, we cannot allow parents to be misled. Babies' health is too important to be left in the hands of a multinational company's marketing department.

> If an ingredient is genuinely found to be beneficial and risk free, then it should be obligatory in all formula milk and not be used as a marketing ploy by a specific brand (de la Torre, 2011, paras 4-6).

EFSA did not make a comparable statement about ARA because "the role of ARA on visual development of term infants cannot be established on the basis of the data presented" (EFSA Panel on Dietetic Products, Nutrition and Allergies, 2009, para 12).

The first DHA-based product intended for infant foods was called Formulaid. In 1994, "The company's pitch to investors has been that Formulaid may help close gaps researchers have found between the development of breast-fed and bottle-fed infants" (Mullaney,

1994, para 4). However, most of the research used as the basis for EFSA's finding in 2011 compares versions of infant formula with and without the additive. The research did not address the question of how infant formulas with DHA compare with breastfeeding, in relation to the development of visual acuity or anything else.

Moreover, the research that was reported used limited, narrow tests of visual acuity. The studies that were cited provide no information about long-term impacts on visual acuity understood broadly.

The health claim supported by EFSA regarding DHA--"DHA contributes to the visual development of infants."--is true, but misleading. The intention was to place that claim on infant formula containers and to use it to promote sales of the product. There is no doubt that DHA as found in breast-milk contributes in important ways to visual development, so in that sense the statement is true. However, that is very different from the claim that some novel synthetic form of DHA blended into infant formula or other infant foods would be effective in the same way as DHA in breast-milk.

As pointed out earlier in the chapter on "How Safe Should Formula Be?" comparisons between different formulas should be distinguished from comparisons between formulas and breast-milk. A health claim that is based on comparisons of the effects on the infant when using different infant formulas should say that. Comparisons of the effects of using those infant formulas with effects of using breast-milk should be explicit about that. This is crucially important in the labeling of any breast-milk substitute. Parents need to make informed choices, not only in deciding which infant formula to use, but also in deciding whether to use formula rather than breastfeed.

The original EFSA approved claim, "DHA contributes to the visual development of infants," was amended in the European Parliament to read, 'Docosahexaenoic acid (DHA) intake contributes to the normal visual development of infants up to 12 months of age" (European Union Register of nutrition and health claims made on food – Authorized health claims, 2011, row 9). That rephrasing does not resolve the inherent ambiguity of the statement.

The European Parliament voted on whether to authorize use of this revised claim on April 6, 2011. The majority of those present voted against it. However, in order to stop the European Commission from authorizing its use, the rules required an absolute majority of all registered members of the Parliament, including the 57 who were not present at the time. Thus, the vote was not strong enough to block this amended claim.

Apart from the confusion regarding the vote count, uncertainties regarding the meaning of the claim were evident. The press release from the European Parliament itself opened by saying:

> Proposals to allow producers to claim that adding the fatty acid DHA to baby food "contributes to the normal visual development of infants up to 12 months of age" were backed by the European Parliament today, when it rejected a move to block them (European Parliament, 2011).

This suggests that the Parliament approved a health claim that said something about adding DHA to baby food. However, the language of the claim that was debated did not say anything about that. And it did not say what type of DHA was under discussion.

The Telegraph newspaper headlined, "EU rules formula milk can claim it is as healthy as breast feeding," which certainly is not the statement that was discussed by the Parliament (Waterfield, 2011).

Baby Milk Action, an advocacy group based in England devoted to "Protecting breastfeeding – Protecting babies fed on formula," mobilized a vigorous campaign against these claims. They argued that the manufacturers' claims about benefits from adding synthetic DHA and ARA to infant formula have been systematically misleading (Baby Milk Action, 2011a, 2011b, 2011c).

The FDA's treatment of additives is different from its approach to food in general (Institute of Medicine, 2004; U.S. Department of Health and Human Services, 2005, 2011d). Its position is that "Companies that want to add new additives to food bear the responsibility of providing FDA with information demonstrating that the additives are safe. FDA experts review the results of appropriate tests done by companies to ensure that the additive is safe for its intended use. . . . Certain food ingredients, such as those with a long history of safe use in food, do not require premarket approval" (U.S. Department of Health and Human Services, 2011d, p. 2).

It is not difficult for food manufacturers to conduct research in which they fail to discover any risks associated with their products.

The debate in Europe over DHA and ARA raised hard questions for the U.S.:

> At the centre of the European debate about DHA Claims are two US companies - Mead Johnson and Martek Biosciences Corporation - who have been in hot water for their eagerness to promote their products. In the US and Canada, there have been private legal actions and investigations by the US **Food and Drug Administration**, the **Federal Trade Commission** and **Health Canada** over their claims, described variously as *'repeated flagrant violation of the US industry self-regulation adjudications'* and as *'unsubstantiated, unacceptable, misleading and unauthorized.'*
>
> . . . The FDA also has serious safety concerns, and in response to a Freedom of Information request from Charlotte Vallaeys of the Cornucopia Institute, in 2007 revealed that it had recorded 98 reports of adverse reactions to DHA fortified formulas. In a letter to Martek, the FDA said: *"some studies have reported adverse events and other morbidities including diarrhea, flatulence, jaundice and apnea in infants fed long-chain polyunsaturated fatty acids"* (Baby Milk Action, 2011b, paras 1, 4).

The U.S. government's safety guidelines with regard to infant formula as set out in 1985 said:

A manufacturer must notify FDA 90 days before the first processing of any infant formula for commercial or charitable distribution for human consumption that differs fundamentally in processing or in composition from any previous formulation produced by the manufacturer (U.S. Department of Health and Human Services, 1985, Section I, para 1).

This means the government is concerned with assessing the effects on safety of any new ingredients that are proposed for infant formula. There is detailed guidance on how these incremental changes are to be assessed (Institute of Medicine, 2004). These are handled by determining whether the proposed additives are GRAS (generally regarded as safe). The FDA often simply accepts the manufacturer's claim regarding the product's safety.

In 2001 the FDA responded to requests from Martek Bioscience Corporation and Mead Johnson Nutritional to have their versions of these fatty acids, ARASCO and DHASCO, characterized as GRAS. In its response, the FDA said:

Based on all of the information provided by Martek, as well as other information available to FDA, the agency has no questions at this time regarding Martek's conclusion that ARASCO and DHASCO are GRAS sources of ARA and DHA under the intended conditions of use - i.e., when added to infant formulas intended for consumption by healthy term infants at a level of up to 1.25 percent each of total dietary fat and at a ratio of DHA to ARA of 1:1 to 1:2. The agency has not, however, made its own determination regarding the GRAS status of the subject use of ARASCO and DHASCO (U.S. Department of Health and Human Services, 2001a, (Conclusions, para 1).

In its similar letter to Mead Johnson Nutritionals, the FDA's conclusion spoke only about ARASCO, and not about DHASCO (U.S. Department of Health and Human Services, 2001b).

These letters said that FDA had no questions about the materials submitted to it about the company's request for GRAS status, and that FDA had not made its own independent determination regarding the GRAS status of the products under discussion. *Neither letter said whether or not FDA agreed with the requests.*

This ambiguous form of language is standard in the FDA's responses to GRAS requests. As one FDA official stated, "FDA responses to GRAS notifications do not constitute FDA approval (U.S. Department of Health and Human Services, 2011g, Section 4). The FDA's Inventory of GRAS Notices website at http://www.fda.gov/Food/FoodIngredientsPackaging/GenerallyRecognizedasSafeGRAS/GRASListings/default.htm shows that the FDA does little more than record the details of the petitions for GRAS that it receives. The FDA does not affirm that the product is safe.

In its letters to both Martek Biosciences Corporation and Mead Johnson Nutritionals, the FDA said:

> FDA would expect any infant formula manufacturer who lawfully markets infant formula containing ARASCO and DHASCO to monitor, through scientific studies and rigorous post-market surveillance, infants who consume such a formula. Importantly, because the broader scientific community could contribute to this continuing evaluation, and because the use of ARASCO and DHASCO in infant formula would be based on the GRAS, provision of the studies would not be considered to be confidential (U.S. Department of Health and Human Services, 2001a, 2001b).

In response to an inquiry from the Cornucopia Institute in 2009, the FDA said it had received no such reports on the safety and effectiveness of these products. Nevertheless, the industry proceeded with large-scale advertising campaigns promoting infant formula and many other food products based on claims about the benefits of these additives (Vallaeys, 2010).

64

It is bad enough that FDA relies on the industry for post-market surveillance of the impacts of new additives. Their value would be highly questionable. It is tragic that the FDA seems indifferent to the failure of the industry to even attempt such studies. Who looks after the interests of the children that might be affected?

The GRAS determination is supposed to be about safety, not about effectiveness, but the two sets of issues have sometimes been mixed together. The differences will be discussed later, in the chapter on "Safety *and* Nutritional Adequacy."

Some people seem to miss the point that GRAS determinations are not about whether particular foods or additives are safe. The GRAS question is about whether they can reasonably be *assumed* to be safe. Why should foods for young children ever be assumed to be safe? That assumption never serves the interests of the children.

The GRAS concept was originally intended as a way to avoid having to scientifically assess familiar products that were known to be safe on the basis of extensive experience in diverse conditions. In the case of novel products, such as synthetic DHA and ARA, intended for highly vulnerable infants, the assumption is absurd on its face. Moreover, there is real division among experts on the benefits of synthetic DHA and ARA to infant formula, and there is evidence of possible harm to infants from these additives (Vallaeys, 2010). Ordinary prudence tells us that the GRAS assumption should not be made. Children should not be burdened with that risk.

These difficulties with additives arise partly because of an anomaly in the current regulation system. Infant formula is sometimes regarded as a standardized commodity, so any product that meets the legal specifications is presumed to be as good as any other. However, product differentiation by brands, advertising, and the stream of different additives imply that some versions of infant formula are superior—even if it is never explicitly acknowledged that others are inferior. It is difficult for consumers to judge the validity of the claims. No independent agency compares different brands.

Labeling practices make it impossible for consumers to determine whether infant formulas contain ingredients that are genetically modified. Some DHA and ARA additives, made on an industrial scale by genetically modified fungi or algae, are claimed to be organic, while others dispute that claim (Vallaeys, 2008). Some critics say the hexane extraction process is particularly hazardous. There has been a great deal of debate over whether additives, such as synthetic DHA and ARA, that are made with solvent extraction processes can be classified as organic (Mitchell, 2011).

The National Organic Program asked the FDA whether DHA and ARA approved for use by FDA as GRAS for infant formula. The FDA offered a convoluted response that basically said their answer was no (U.S. Department of Health and Human Services, 2011g, Note 5). Current regulations do not say the labels must reveal that these are novel microbial oils produced by industrial processes. As historian Maureen Minchin has said, "Such regulatory decisions do not seem to have informed parental choice as their prime object, and certainly assist industry" (M. Minchin, personal communication, 2011).

There are many infant formulas on the market that claim to be organic, but given the obscurity of the rules, the meaning and validity of those claims remain unclear.

There is a website (www.storebrandformula.com) that argues, "There are no better formulas. Only more expensive ones." Other websites offer similar claims (Baby Center, 2011). If it is true that there are no formulas that are better than the ones that meet the basic requirements for infant formula set out in the 1980s, why do many manufacturers offer additives?

At one time Wyeth Nutrition made most of the generic or "store brand" formulas sold in the U.S., but now PBM products makes them. PBM was purchased by Perrigo in 2010.

In the U.S.,

> The infant formula market is highly concentrated. In 2008, three manufacturers accounted for 98 percent of all dollar sales. Abbott (43 percent) and Mead Johnson (40 percent) accounted for the bulk of dollar sales, while Nestlé accounted for another 15 percent. Most of the remaining two percent of infant formula sales were accounted for by PBM Nutritionals, producer of the Bright Beginnings line of infant formulas, as well as private-label or storebrand formulas (Oliveria & Smallwood, 2010, p. 6).

It should not be assumed that health is the primary concern of those who promote additives in infant formula. In the 1990s, a Hambricht & Quist Spot Report recommending stocks highlighted Martek Biosciences and its new Formulaid, a blend of DHA and ARA. The stock promotion said:

> Infant formula is currently a commodity market, with all products being almost identical and marketers competing intensely to differentiate their product. Even if Formulaid had no benefit, we think that it would be widely incorporated into most formulas as a marketing tool and to allow companies to promote their formula as 'closest to human milk' (INFACT Canada, 1997, Fools Gold: Recommendation-Strong Buy).

The marketers of infant formula are clear about the benefits to the industry of product differentiation. To illustrate:

> The 2010 launch of Materna Extra Care is expected to boost sales of premium products in milk formula and also alter the quality of standard milk formula in Israel. The new launch also brought to Israel the new global trend of powder milk formula that is as close as possible to human breast-milk, and this trend

is expected to continue having a significant impact on both manufacturers and parents throughout the forecast period. In 2010, the Israeli Ambulatory Pediatric Association, in collaboration with the Ministry of Health, launched a new report stating that powder milk formula should contain LU-PUFA and iron in order to best promote infant development. A rise is therefore expected in the quality of the products and brands of the leading baby food players over the forecast period as new product launches bring added value, better infant nutrition and higher quality (Euromonitor International, 2010, para 3).

Claiming that Formulaid is "closest to human milk" or that Materna Extra Care is "as close as possible to human milk" is a bit like claiming that New York is closer to Paris than New Jersey is to Paris. That may be true, but the difference is minor when compared to the great distance of both of them from Paris.

Additives have led to rapid increases in infant formula prices throughout the world despite the scientific uncertainties regarding their claimed benefits for the children. According to Maureen Minchin, "Most parents in affluent countries are prepared to pay for the most expensive formula option, assuming this means they are getting the best alternative to breast-milk. The use of the word "gold" on the labels of additive-enhanced formulas has been allowed to go unchecked" (M. Minchin, personal communication, 2011). Using "gold" to describe any infant formula is misleading when breastfeeding is really the gold standard when it comes to ensuring children's health.

Some people say that if an additive can be clearly shown to be beneficial, without simultaneously resulting in significant harm, it should be added to the list of required ingredients for infant formula. Rather than regard it as optional and perhaps have it available only to high-income families, all formula-fed infants should get it. A great deal of good research would have to be done to determine that a proposed new component should be required in all infant formula.

Some analysts suggest that DHA and ARA additives might be appropriate for some infants with unusual needs, but not for the great majority of infants (Heinig et al., 2010). Infant formulas for infants with those needs could be distributed on a prescription basis, rather than through commercial marketing.

A useful website for tracking reports on additives in infant formula and other foods is available at www.nutraingredients.com. The reports are diverse, but generally seem more concerned with market shares than with health impacts.

Product differentiation of branded infant formula based on additives and advertising systematically leads to increased costs to consumers, but with little evidence of health benefits for most infants. New additives can introduce new risks of harm. These are not only national or regional issues; they are global. They should be addressed at the global level, with priority given to ensuring that modifications to infant formula promote infant health and cause no significant harm.

ISSUE 6.	The value of additives to infant formulas should be assessed through sound scientific procedures. They should not be assumed to be safe and effective.

8 | Safety *and* Nutritional Adequacy

Codex Alimentarius recognizes a wide range of contaminants of infant formula (Codex Alimentarius Commission, 2008). The European Food Safety Authority is very attentive to such risks. China, having gone through widely publicized contamination issues, is now very sensitive to the need to ensure the safety of infant formula (PR Newswire, 2011). The United States' Food and Drug Administration provides regular information on infant formula safety problems, such as *Enterobacter sakazakii* infection outbreaks (U.S. Department of Health and Human Services, 2011a). The agency also provides information on infant formula that has been recalled and on blocked imports. All this attention reinforces people's confidence that governments are ensuring the quality of infant formula.

However, there is an old saying: A ship in the harbor is safe, but that is not what it is for. Apart from being safe, there are things that ships are supposed to do. Similarly, we expect more from infant formula than merely being safe. Governments have focused on infant formula's safety, not its nutritional adequacy. Governments should give more attention to what infant formula is supposed to do.

Pharmaceuticals are assessed for both their safety and their effectiveness. Safety is about ensuring the product does no harm in the short term. Effectiveness is about ensuring that it does what it is supposed to do, its functionality. For example, if a claim is made that a product will reduce fever, it should be demonstrated scientifically that it does in fact accomplish that. Pharmaceuticals are expected to carry out certain functions effectively. Much of the trouble with infant formula traces to the fact that not enough has been done to ensure its effectiveness, its nutritional adequacy.

Infant formula is not officially a pharmaceutical product, though in many cases the manufacturers are pharmaceutical companies. They do not make explicit claims about effectiveness, so it is difficult to fault them on that dimension. However, there is an implicit claim that infant formula can be regarded as a close approximation to breast-milk in terms of its functionality. The United States Code defines infant formula as "a food that purports to be or is represented for special dietary use solely as a food for infants by reason of its simulation of human milk."

To say that infant formula is safe in the sense that it has no *E. Coli* bacteria in it or that it includes all the ingredients in a prescribed list is different from saying that it has all the elements that contribute to living a long and healthy life. Saying that a food won't make you sick right away is not the same as saying that it meets your needs. Short-term food safety is not the only thing that matters.

The designation of a food as GRAS depends on whether it is judged to be safe, not on whether it is nutritionally adequate. The GRAS concept does not require any assessment of whether the food is functionally effective. Where food safety assessments limit their attention to things like contaminants and adverse events, equal attention should be given to nutritional adequacy. What does the product do for the human being who consumes it?

The U.S. Food and Drug Administration explicitly states that it does not approve functional claims for foods (U.S. Department of Health and Human Services, 2011d). Thus it will not address claims that particular infant formulas help infants to grow or to have good eyesight. *There is no agency that ensures the functional quality of infant formula.*

The main function of infant food and the associated feeding process is to ensure long-term health–including not only body-building, but also protection against infections and allergies, and facilitating cognitive as well as physical development. The only way to ensure that feeding with any breast-milk substitute is closely equivalent to breastfeeding would be to compare the health of children who are breastfed with the health of those who use the substitute. Health status should be assessed not only in the short term, but also in the long term.

Explicit standards for functionality have been considered. In the discussion leading up to the adoption of 21 CFR Parts 106 and 107, the rules relating to infant formula in the U.S., there was a proposal requiring that "formula will support optimal infant growth and health" The proposal said, "FDA has tentatively concluded, therefore that an evaluation of the ability of a formula to support healthy growth must be made under its most demanding conditions of use, i.e., when it is used as the sole source of nutrition." It also said, "the determination of physical growth rate is the most valuable component of the clinical evaluation of infant formulas" (U.S. Federal Register, 1996, pp. 36157, 36180). However, this recognition of the importance of physical growth did not carry over into the rules that were finally adopted.

Although there are issues regarding the precise relationship between infant growth and health (De Onis, Garza, Victora, Bhan, & Norum, 2004; Fomon, 2004; Garza & de Onis, 1999), there is clear consensus that healthy infants grow rapidly (but not too rapidly) and have low rates of morbidity and mortality. International agencies have worked out clear standards for normal growth rates of infants and young children.

Current regulations for infant formula focus on ensuring that particular components are supplied in specified quantities, based on an ingredients list from the 1980s. They assume that any formula that includes the specified ingredients in the required amounts is safe and nutritionally adequate. However, breast-milk is a complex, changing, living thing, and not simply a collection of inert ingredients. The ingredients in the list are different in form from those in breast-milk

(Packard, 1982). This list does not take into account the fact that the composition of breast-milk changes as the child matures. Infant formula cannot mimic that incremental adaptation process.

The complexity is illustrated by the fact that iron in breast-milk is readily available (bioavailable) to the child, but it is not readily available in infant formula. Thus, some manufacturers have included much higher levels of iron in formula than is found in breast-milk. The result can be toxic in various ways (Lönnerdal & Kelleher, 2007).

Feeding infants with formula regularly leads to worse health outcomes than are obtained with breastfeeding. Sometimes they are much worse, sometimes not. This inferiority in terms of functions is not surprising, since the structure of infant formula is very different from the structure of breast-milk. The contrast is indicated by the images in Figure 8.1.

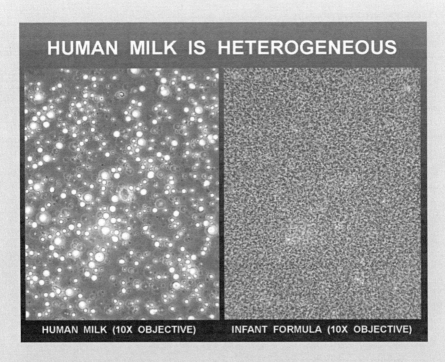

Figure 8.1. Breast-milk and Infant Formula.

Source: Stephen Buescher, Professor of Pediatrics, Eastern Virginia Medical School, Norfolk, Virginia. Used with permission.

The image on the left shows a natural product, while the one on the right looks like an undifferentiated industrial product.

The claim that infant formula is both safe and effective (nutritionally adequate) if it includes a basic list of ingredients is a simplistic, reductionist approach, treating something very complex as if it were the same as the sum of its components. Who would look at an exquisite painting and suggest it is nothing more than reds, greens, and blues, or that a piano concerto can be conveyed by listing the musical notes? Who would describe a meal prepared by an excellent chef simply in terms of its ingredients? To suggest that one can approximate breast-milk by putting a few ingredients into a mixer is to grossly underestimate it.

This reductionist approach has dangerous consequences. As nutritionist Carlos Monteiro explains:

> Nutrition science is taught and practiced as a biochemical discipline. Practically all nutritionists now categorise food in terms of its chemical composition, as do most lay writers. This almost universal perception of nutrition is evident in textbooks and scientific journals, and on food labels, journalism, and 'diet books'. The identification of food with its chemistry is a defining characteristic of modern nutrition science, as invented in the early 19th century. Seeing food in terms of its chemistry has enabled the industrialisation of food systems. In particular, it has made possible the formulation of ultra-processed products from 'refined' or 'purified' chemical constituents of foods – oils, proteins, carbohydrates, and their fractions – together with 'micronutrients' – vitamins and minerals (Monteiro, 2011, p. 87).

He summarizes: "Identification of food mainly with its chemical constituents at best has limited value, and in general has proved to be unhelpful, misleading, and harmful to public health" (Monteiro, 2011, p. 87).

The Codex *Statement on Infant Formula* of 1976 said, "Numerous formulae have been produced which offer a nutritionally adequate food for infants . . ." (Codex Alimentarius Commission, 1976, para 3). Of course that depends on how one understands "nutritionally adequate." Elsewhere *Codex Alimentarius* says:

> The nutritional adequacy of a product can be defined in terms of protein quality and quantity and content of minerals and vitamins.
>
> Such a product should be considered nutritionally equivalent if:
>
> i. its protein quality is not less than that of the original product or is equivalent to that of casein and
>
> ii. it contains the equivalent quantity of protein (N 6.25) and those vitamins and minerals which are present in significant amounts in the original animal products (Codex Alimentarius Commission, 1989, Section 7.2).

This is difficult to understand. A food's nutritional adequacy should be assessed in terms of its results, not its ingredients. Infant formula should be viewed as nutritionally adequate only if it is proven to be as good for children as breastfeeding. Any other definition shortchanges children.

Infant formula products should be assessed on the basis of their safety and their nutritional adequacy. Assessing them on the basis of their safety and their composition (as in Crawley & Westland, 2011) is a serious error. A study that focuses almost exclusively on the composition of infant formula is of little help in assessing the risks involved in its use.

There is value to checking the composition of infant formula because it can deteriorate over time, it may be manufactured improperly, and it may be contaminated in various ways. Thus, it is good to know that the China Dairy Industry Association is testing samples on a monthly basis, especially in light of the tragic history of contaminated Chinese-made infant formula. However, they will only test formula from those dairy enterprises that voluntarily apply to be part of the program. It is not clear exactly what tests will be made. A Chinese dairy industry expert "called for government to take on a stronger role in policing the industry, because having industry associations regulate the industry could lead to conflicts of interest" (Crienglish, 2011, para 5).

Even perfect adherence to imperfect recipes for infant formula puts infants at risk.

Contrary to Codex's 1976 claim that, "Numerous formulae have been produced which offer a nutritionally adequate food for infants," (Codex Alimentarius Commission, 1976, para 3), *there has never been any infant formula that is nutritionally adequate.*

If any infant formula that meets a specific list of required ingredients is nutritionally adequate, how would we explain why so many different infant formula products are available on the market? In the United Kingdom alone one can obtain:

- Infant milks suitable from birth (cows' milk based)
- Infant milks marketed for hungrier babies, suitable from birth (cows' milk based)
- Thickened infant milks suitable from birth
- Soy protein based infant milks suitable from birth
- Lactose-free infant milks suitable from birth
- Partially hydrolyzed infant milks suitable from birth

And for older infants one can obtain:

- Follow-on formula suitable from six months of age
- Partially hydrolyzed follow-on formula suitable from six months of age
- Goodnight milks and food drinks

- Food drink

- Growing-up milks and toddler milks (Crawley & Westland, 2011)

Many new varieties are offered all the time, including those discussed earlier in the chapter on Additives.

In 1981, Codex said, "Infant formula means a breast-milk substitute specially manufactured to satisfy, by itself, the nutritional requirements of infants during the first months of life up to the introduction of appropriate complementary feeding" (Codex Alimentarius Commission, 2007, Section 2.1.1, p. 1). If we assess formula by its results, rather than by whether its ingredients matched a specific list, there has never been an infant formula that would "satisfy, by itself, the nutritional requirements of infants during the first months of life."

The European Union has said that, "Infant formula is the only processed foodstuff which wholly satisfies the nutritional requirements of infants during the first months of life until the introduction of appropriate complementary feeding" (EUR-Lex, 2011, para 4; also see Article 2(c) and Article 3). The statement should be rejected. If infant formula *wholly* satisfied infants' requirements, there would not be a regular pattern of worse health outcomes for infants who use it.

The industry's lobbying group based in the U.S., the Infant Formula Council, says, "Standard iron-fortified baby formulas are nutritionally complete foods for normal infants" (Infant Formula Council, 2011, Frequently Asked Questions/What Nutrients are Present in Infant Formula and Why Are They Included?, para 2). One possible interpretation of "nutritionally complete" is that the formulas comply with the list of required ingredients under the law. If they are complete, why do the manufacturers offer additives beyond those required by the law? If nutritionally adequate infant formula had already been developed by the 1980s, why has there been a steady stream of additives since then?

Perhaps the Infant Formula Council means to say that the formulas are complete in the sense that they meet all infants' nutritional needs. If that is the position, then how would they explain the consistently worse health outcomes with formula feeding when compared with breastfeeding? Either way, the claim that infant formulas are "nutritionally complete" is misleading.

The Infant Nutrition Council based in Australia makes a claim similar to the one by the Infant Formula Council in the U.S.: "Infant formula has been specifically developed to contain all the necessary ingredients needed to meet an infant's nutritional requirements" (Infant Nutrition Council, 2011, Formula Information/Frequently Asked Questions/2). How is infant formula the only suitable substitute to breast-milk?). If formula has *all* the ingredients needed to meet nutritional requirements, why add things? And how would they explain the fact that formula feeding leads to worse health outcomes than breastfeeding?

When the World Health Organization investigated the adequacy of exclusive breastfeeding during the first six months of infants' lives, the study focused not on the composition of the diet, but on its results:

> In evaluating the nutrient adequacy of exclusive breastfeeding, infant nutrient requirements are assessed in terms of relevant functional outcomes. Nutrient adequacy is most commonly evaluated in terms of growth, but other functional outcomes, e.g., immune response and neurodevelopment, are also considered to the extent that available data permit.
> . . .
>
> In determining the optimal duration of exclusive breastfeeding in specific contexts, it is important that functional outcomes, e.g., infant morbidity and mortality, also are taken into consideration (Butte, Lopez-Alarcon, & Garza, 2002, p. vii).

Other kinds of feeding methods could be studied by examining their impacts on these outcome indicators. The common standards would make it possible to compare the nutritional adequacy of different methods of feeding.

Given the heavy influence of the infant formula industry in Codex, European, and FDA deliberations, the weakness of the standards for infant formula is not surprising (Koletzko & Shamir, 2006; Palmer, 2009). As Elisabeth Sterken of INFACT Canada put it:

> The FAO/WHO *Codex Alimentarius* standard setting process may be one of the best examples of how the governments of infant formula producing countries protect the formula industries. The US, German, Dutch, Swiss, Japanese governments, and the EC consistently promote standard setting that deregulates as much as they can ethically get away with.
>
> Just to give a few examples:
>
> 1. The approval of higher levels of added nutrients is based on "history of use," not rigorous science to prove safety and efficacy. This is to accommodate marketing needs: i.e., longer shelf life under as many environmental conditions as possible and the new preparation guidelines which will instruct parents to mix powdered formulas with water previously boiled and then cooled to 70 degrees Celcius. Preparation at these temperatures risks destroying some of the heat labile nutrients and increasing levels of ammonia, furfurals, etc. However this temperature is needed to reduce the risk of infection by *E sakazakii*. The industry is not being mandated to have zero tolerance for *E sakazakii*.
>
> 2. The refusal to require warnings on powdered infant formulas that the product is not sterile and

may contain pathogenic microorganisms. The only reason for this is to protect the industry - claiming that warning labels would "scare" parents. Without a warning as to the rationale for the proposed rigorous preparation instructions, it will be difficult for parents to follow them. However, the blame will, of course, fall on the parents if something goes wrong because they will not have followed the manufacturers' instructions. Shifting blame reduces liability for the industry. Throughout the draft for the Code of Hygienic practice for powdered formulas, the emphasis is on caregivers having to follow instructions. Canada tried very hard to reduce the scope of this standard to only "high risk" infants less than two months of age, thus eliminating formulas for infants older than two months from having to comply with risk reduction recommendations for pathogenic microorganisms.

3. Nutrition and health claims are used in a very aggressive way by the industry without accepted scientific validation for these claims. Comparisons are made with other formulas or cow's milk, yet the product promos give the impression that this gives the product breast-milk equality. Governments wink at these deceptions and the industry keeps the research "confused." Codex went through all kinds of delays and hoops to keep the standards from fully restricting nutrition and health claims. We did achieve some restrictions, but this must also be done at the national level to be effective. So for many countries if national legislation does not prohibit claims, then the imports from producing countries will have claims - on labels in advertisements, brochures etc....in countries where the impact of all this is deadly.

4. Industry is always present and very available with funding for "government delegations." For example, at the Working Group to draft the standard for the code

of hygienic practice for powdered formulas, the Swiss delegate was a Nestle employee. At all Codex meetings dealing with infant formula standards, government delegations are sprinkled with representatives from the industry. The process rules should, of course, disallow such blatant conflict of interest, but it is up to the member states to change the rules and, of course, there is no will or consensus to do this. The determination of venues and chairpersons are also key in protecting industry interests. Germany, as the host country for the standard setting for infant formulas, has for years appointed a chair with clear links to the industry.

I can go on with more examples. My point in all this is the resistance to regulate formula quality and labeling comes from governments surrounded by legions of industry lobbyists and is at the expense of human health. And the Codex Alimentarius is a key global instrument to achieve this (E. Sterken, personal communication, 2006).

The industry lobbies to keep the standards weak, with the result that infants are exposed to excessive risks. The industry lobbyists accept the statement that breastfeeding is best, but they resist statements that say formula feeding is worse. They do not talk about the types and degrees of risk associated with formula feeding when compared with breastfeeding (Democracy Now, 2005; Petersen, 2003; Ross & Rackmill, 2004). They do not encourage the collection of data needed to analyze the risks of using infant formula in comparison with breastfeeding.

Governments and the formula industry have different interests and responsibilities in relation to infant formula. The companies' fiduciary obligation to their stockholders is to maximize their profits, within the law. They might compromise on other dimensions. In this context, the primary concern of governments should be the wellbeing of infants and their families.

Perhaps they key pivotal element in this context is the profession committed to child health–the pediatricians. If they throw their weight to the side of the industry, that greatly limits the capacity of government to create and enforce effective regulations in support of infants and their families. It is no surprise that the formula industry spends a great deal of money on cultivating the favor of pediatricians.

So long as feeding with infant formula consistently produces worse health outcomes than breastfeeding in every sort of population, formula should not be viewed as nutritionally adequate. Feeding with formula might be claimed to be good enough for some purposes, but it should never be said or implied to be as good, or nearly as good, as breastfeeding.

Parents might have valid reasons for feeding their children with something that is not as good as breastfeeding. They should never be misled into believing it is almost as good.

ISSUE 7.	Standards for infant formula should require demonstration of nutritional adequacy as well as safety

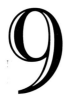

Distribution of Formula by Governments

There are serious issues regarding the distribution of infant formula by national governments and international agencies.

The idea of sending infant formula into disaster situations has been questioned, as illustrated in Kim Hekimian Arzoumanian's account of the experience following the 1988 earthquake in Armenia:

> Formula was solicited and distributed after the earthquake on the faulty premise that the nutrition provided by breast-milk is somehow inadequate. Arzoumanian found, however, that the real problems lie with infant formula. One problem was that people sometimes used impure water to dilute the formula. This practice led to infant diarrhea and other morbidities.
>
> Another problem lay in the simple fact that unlike milk, formula had to be acquired from sources not under the mother's control. According to Arzoumanian, the free distribution of four-to-six-week supplies of formula got untold numbers of mothers hooked. Fresh supplies were not always available, however,

and mothers would run out of formula. By then they had stopped lactating and had no nutritious and appropriate way to feed their infants (Armenian Forum, 1998, paras 5-6).

This and similar experiences elsewhere have led to stringent limitations on the provision of infant formula in emergency situations (Gribble, McGrath, Maclaine, & Lhotska, 2011; Wellstart International, 2005; World Health Organization, 2007b).

Concerns also arise around the fact that several national governments regularly distribute infant formula at no or low cost, usually to people with low-incomes. For example, Britain's Healthy Start program provides vouchers that can be exchanged for various foods, including infant formula. Women with low incomes can get vouchers valued at £3.10 every week if they are pregnant, £6.20 a week for each child under the age of one, and £3.10 a week for each child between the ages of one and four.

When a Member of Parliament asked the Secretary of State for Health about why infant formula is on the list of acceptable foods, she was told, "We recommend exclusive breastfeeding for the first six months of life, and the scheme encourages this. However, if mothers choose not to breastfeed, formula is the only safe alternative for children under one year of age, as the use of cow's milk is not recommended" (NCT Watch, 2009, para 2). Women may use the vouchers for infant formula, but they may use them for other groceries as well.

The United Kingdom also has a scheme for distributing infant formula in daycare centers. Pamela Morrison, an international board certified lactation consultant, voiced her concerns about it to a Member of Parliament:

> It seems that there is a scheme in place, administered by the Department of Health in England and on behalf of the devolved administrations in Scotland and Wales, which enables registered day care providers (child minders, crèches and nurseries) to obtain free

dried baby milk for babies under 12 months who are in their care for two hours or more per day. Day care providers who have been approved to supply milk under the scheme can be reimbursed the cost of the milk they supply. It is called Nursery Milk Reimbursement Unit (see http://www.nurserymilk. co.uk/).

As we know it is often perceived by healthcare providers that it is too difficult for working mothers to provide their own expressed milk for their babies when they return to work, so that there is little point in an employed mother attempting to maintain breastfeeding. It's such a pity, because it's actually quite easy - it simply takes high motivation, and some careful planning. And the results are so worthwhile because of course breastfed babies remain healthier so that benefits accrue to babies, mothers and employers, and the NHS in reduced healthcare costs. I've worked with employed mothers of even young babies who have exclusively breastfed during the hours when they are at home with their babies, and exclusively breast-milk-fed when separated from them for work or school. Once the babies start solid foods (after six months) then it becomes even easier to continue breastfeeding early mornings, evenings and during the night, and the baby can have other foods at daycare.

It is hard to believe that no-one can appreciate that the provision of free formula milk at daycare would further deter a working mother from making the extra effort to leave her own milk for her baby. When the Department of Health endorses formula-feeding and provides formula for free, why should she bother? The easy access to free formula would also no doubt influence the day care provider to trivialize the value (and safety?) of breast-milk should a mother plan to leave it for the baby while she works. Nevertheless, not only is the baby suffering from this provision of "free" formula milk which undermines his health and nutrition, but valuable tax-payer pounds are being wasted in subsidising private daycare nurseries and potentially parents who can well afford to feed their children themselves. Government is effectively subsidizing the formula industry, which not only goes against the spirit and aim of the *International Code of Marketing of Breast-Milk Substitutes* and subsequent World Health Assembly resolutions ... but lends its seal of approval to a feeding method known to cause more infection, allergy, obesity and sub-optimal cognitive development, compared to breast-milk (P. Morrison, personal communication, 2011).

The *International Code of Marketing of Breast-Milk Substitutes* does not directly address the issue of formula distribution by governments. It is primarily concerned with the actions of infant formula manufacturers, and views governments mainly in their role as regulators of those manufacturers. However, there is no reason to doubt that, as Morrison suggests, distribution of infant formula by governments goes against the spirit and aim of the Code.

The U.S. government distributes free infant formula on a larger scale than any other country through its Special Supplemental Nutrition Program for Women, Infants, and Children, commonly known as WIC. Its mission is "To safeguard the health of low-income women, infants, and children up to age 5 who are at nutrition risk by providing nutritious foods to supplement diets, information on healthy eating, and referrals to health care" (WIC, 2011a, para 1). It is managed under detailed federal laws and regulations (WIC, 2011b). WIC's requirements for standard infant formula are as follows:

- Complies with the definition in section 201(z) of the Federal Food, Drug and Cosmetic Act (21 U.S.C. 321(z)) and meets the requirements for an infant formula under section 412 of the Federal Food, Drug Act (21 U.S.C. 350a) and regulations at 21 CFR Parts 106 and 107.

- Nutritionally complete infant formula not requiring the addition of any ingredients other than water prior to being served in a liquid state.

- Be designed for enteral digestion via an oral or tube feeding.

- Provide at least 10 mg iron per liter (at least 1.8 mg iron/100 kilocalories) at standard dilution.

- Provide at least 67 kilocalories per 100 milliliters (approximately 20 kilocalories per fluid ounce) at standard dilution.

The requirements for "exempt" infant formula, for infants with particular needs are different:

- Complies with the definition and requirements for an exempt infant formula in section 412(h) of the Federal Food, Drug and Cosmetic Act (21U.S.C. 350a(h)) and regulations at 21 CFR Parts 106 and 107.

- Be designed for enteral digestion via an oral or tube feeding.

- Requires medical documentation for issuance.

About half of all infants in the U.S. participate in the WIC program (Oliveira, Frazão, & Smallwood, 2010). In December 2010, the program was recorded as serving 8,870,000 participants, and providing an average monthly benefit worth $43.22 (U.S Department of Agriculture, Food and Nutrition Service, 2010).

WIC serves families under the official poverty line and also low-income families, defined by WIC as those under 185 percent of the poverty line. In addition, women and children in families that are eligible for or are receiving benefits from certain other federal programs are categorically eligible for WIC services. The program serves children up to the age of five. Women who request infant formula can receive it only up to the child's first birthday.

In 2004-2006, 57-68 percent of all infant formula used in the U.S. was provided through the WIC program, at no cost to the families. About 88 percent of the infants in WIC receive some infant formula from the program (Oliveira et al., 2010). Since about half the infants in the US receive WIC services, about 44 percent of U.S. infants obtain formula through WIC.

While WIC clearly helps to improve the health of its participants, there is debate about the wisdom of its large-scale distribution of infant formula. In providing infant formula through WIC, the U.S. government can be seen as promoting excessive formula use (Kent, 2006). This goes against the breastfeeding advocacy of other government agencies, such as the U.S. Centers for Disease Control and Prevention (2010) and the U.S. Department of Health and Human Services (2010a, 2010b). It also goes against the advice of non-governmental agencies, such as the National Alliance for Breastfeeding Advocacy and the U.S. Breastfeeding Committee. WIC's large-scale distribution of infant formula is contrary to the principles set out in the *International Code of Marketing of Breast-Milk Substitutes.*

It has been estimated that the added healthcare and related costs in the U.S. associated with not breastfeeding are about $13 billion a year (Bartick & Reinhold, 2010). A comparable analysis shows that formula feeding in Britain costs the government millions of pounds for healthcare (NICE, 2006). The methodology and the exact conclusions of these studies are open to dispute, but the general finding, that formula use results in high healthcare and other costs, is beyond dispute. Reducing the amount of formula provided by WIC in the U.S. or by Healthy Start in Britain would reduce overall costs to the government. If healthcare and other related costs were taken into account, governments might not be so willing to provide infant formula through their programs. If healthcare costs that were paid by agencies outside WIC were internalized by the program, it probably would make different policy decisions.

A similar argument could be made with regard to mothers' decision-making process. If they had to bear the full cost of infant formula and also the added healthcare costs that might be associated with its use, they might make different choices. They might be making distorted choices because they are insulated from these costs by government agencies.

If government agencies stopped providing infant formula altogether, some women might feed with seriously inadequate breast-milk substitutes, such as cow's milk. Women who chose to purchase formula on their own might over-dilute it to save money. These actions could increase health problems and healthcare costs. However, strong educational programs could help to minimize these problems. Presumably, there is an optimum somewhere between large-scale formula distribution and zero formula distribution that would maximize health and minimize healthcare costs.

WIC has been doing a great deal to promote breastfeeding, including redesigning its food packages to strengthen the incentive for women to choose to breastfeed (Institute of Medicine, 2005). In some states, such as California, WIC has taken strong initiatives to promote breastfeeding, resulting in a decline in participants' requests for infant formula. One observer explained the six percent decrease in formula sales in the U.S. in 2010 by saying, "A slowdown in birth rates, a trend towards breastfeeding, and a change in the WIC programme contributed to reduced sales of milk formula" (Euromonitor International, 2011, Trends).

The USDA analyzed the national impacts of the new food package on the quantity of infant formula used in the WIC program:

> The results show that the total quantity prescribed under the new food package is about 20 percent smaller than the quantity prescribed under the old food package. Reductions in infant formula use are observed across most age and feeding methods.

However,

> Fully formula-fed infants four to five months of age are the only group where infant formula use is higher under the new food package than under the old food package (Oliveira et al., 2010, p. 37).

A study of the impacts of the new WIC food package in Texas showed small decreases in formula consumption for most age groups of infants, and small increases for those who were 11 months old (Murano et al., 2011, Slide 63).

WIC's breastfeeding promotion efforts are good, but not likely to be of the scale needed. It would take a much larger effort to counteract the strong incentive effect of offering free name-brand infant formula that appears to be endorsed by government (Tuttle, 2000; Kent, 2006).

WIC could adopt the system used in Britain's Healthy Start program. Women get vouchers of specific cash value that can be used for formula, regular milk, or other sorts of groceries. The program does not provide any distinct incentive to use infant formula.

Careful monitoring of health outcomes and healthcare costs could help WIC and similar programs in other countries to safeguard health more effectively. Analyses that showed the relationship between different methods of feeding and healthcare costs would help in assessing the economic impacts of the program's policy on families and also on the government.

In the 1990s, studies showed that the WIC program was effective in reducing child mortality, improving children's health, and reducing their healthcare costs, especially their Medicaid costs (e.g., GAO, 1992; Devaney & Schrim, 1993). Similar studies could be done to estimate the impacts of different methods of feeding.

WIC has become concerned about the effectiveness and the costs of additives to infant formula. As pointed out earlier, few of the additives have been assessed adequately to determine whether they provide the claimed benefits (California WIC Association, 2010; True, 2011). The cost increases have been significant:

> All rebate contracts in effect in December 2008 were based on formulas supplemented with the fatty acids docosahexaenoic acid (DHA) and arachidonic

acid (ARA), whereas most of the previous contracts were based on unsupplemented formulas. Because wholesale prices of DHA/ARA-supplemented formulas are higher than wholesale prices of unsupplemented formulas, wholesale prices of infant formula increased more in States that switched to the more expensive DHA/ARA-supplemented formula in their contracts that were in effect in December 2008 (Oliveira et al., 2010, pp. iii-iv).

According to the nongovernmental Center on Budget & Policy Priorities, "WIC appears to be spending more than $90 million extra annually–or more than ten percent of its total spending on infant formula–to provide formulas with ingredients that neither USDA nor the FDA has assessed with regard to their benefits" (Neuberger 2010a, p. 6). Thus it makes no sense to have "WIC spend extra taxpayer funds on products with functional ingredients without considering whether scientific evidence demonstrates that they have health or developmental benefits" (Neuberger, 2010a, p. 13; also see Neuberger 2010b).

The seemingly endless stream of new additives leads to steady inflation of the price of infant formula. "Thus, a troubling and costly cycle is beginning to affect WIC's bottom line, in which the 'designer' formulas that carry higher wholesale (and retail) prices become the standard, increasing WIC costs and requiring Congress to appropriate more funds for WIC to pay for them" (California WIC Association 2010, p. 3). Why does WIC pay higher prices for supplemented formula if there is no good evidence of nutritional or other benefits?

The procurement issues discussed in the following chapter are relevant. Procurement policies can significantly impact the health and economic impacts of governmental programs for the distribution of infant formula.

One has to wonder about the seriousness of the U.S. government's efforts to promote breastfeeding when the *HHS Blueprint for Action on Breastfeeding* published in 2000 failed to mention WIC's program for the distribution of infant formula (U.S. Department of Health and Human Services, 2000). The Surgeon General's *Call to Action to Support Breastfeeding* in 2011 also failed to take notice of it (U.S. Department of Health and Human Services, 2011b).

Despite many indications that feeding with infant formula increases the likelihood of children being overweight, First Lady Michelle Obama's well-funded child obesity program gives little attention to infant feeding practices and the role of WIC. The Institute of Medicine's study on Early Childhood Obesity Prevention Policies acknowledged, "there is an association between breastfeeding and a reduction in obesity risk," and cited several studies in support of that point (Birch, Parker, & Burns, 2011, p. 4-2). However, it did not explicitly say that infant formula might be a factor leading to overweight in children, and it did not mention WIC's formula distribution program.

The California WIC Association, a nongovernmental group that supports the WIC program in California, has given a good deal of attention to the issue of overweight children (Whaley et al., 2010). However, it has focused on things like food and beverage intake, and physical activity. Apparently, it has not looked into the possibility that WIC's distribution of infant formula might be a significant contributor to overweight in children.

While U.S. government agencies do many good things to support breastfeeding and to prevent overweight in children, it seems that questioning WIC's provision of infant formula is somehow off limits.

ISSUE 8.	Government agencies should limit the provision of infant formula or any other foods that place children at significant risk regarding their health.

10 Procurement Policies

Government programs that distribute infant formula have various policies for procuring the product for their participants. The arrangements in the WIC program are distinctive, but some of the concerns may be relevant for other programs as well.

WIC's system is summarized as follows:

> USDA's Special Supplemental Nutrition Program for Women, Infants, and Children (WIC) provides participating infants with free infant formula. Federal law requires that WIC State agencies enter into cost-containment contracts with infant formula manufacturers, with agencies typically receiving substantial discounts (rebates) from manufacturers for each can of formula purchased through the program. Each WIC State agency or group of agencies awards a contract to the manufacturer offering the lowest net wholesale price, defined as the difference between the manufacturer's wholesale price and the rebate. In exchange for the rebate, a manufacturer is given an exclusive right to provide its infant formula to WIC participants in the State. In fiscal 2008, infant formula rebates totaled $2.0 billion, compared with

total WIC expenditures (after rebates) of $6.2 billion (Oliveira et al., 2010, p. iii).

Figure 10.1 helps to explain the concepts:

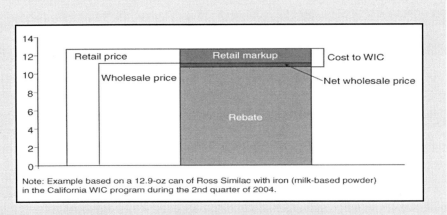

Note: Example based on a 12.9-oz can of Ross Similac with iron (milk-based powder) in the California WIC program during the 2nd quarter of 2004.

Figure 10.1. Cost components for can of infant formula in WIC (dollars per can).

Source: Oliveira, V., Frazão, E., & Smallwood, D. (2010). *Rising infant formula costs to the WIC Program: Recent trends in rebates and wholesale prices.* Washington, D.C.: U.S. Department of Agriculture. http://www.ers.usda.gov/Publications/ERR93/

The procurement rules are spelled out in the *U.S. Code of Federal Regulations* at 7CFR246.16a.

Several difficulties with this system could affect both the quality and the cost of the product that is obtained.

One concern is that the requirement of competitive bidding limits WIC's opportunity to evaluate alternative products. WIC regulations simply require that the product includes the prescribed list of ingredients,. The procurement regulations do not allow for assessment of product quality in all its dimensions.

A second issue is that the small number of bidders raises questions about possible monopolistic practices. Over the last decade only three manufacturers have bid for WIC contracts: Mead Johnson (Enfamil), Abbott (Similac), and Nestlé (Good Start Supreme) (Oliveira et al., 2010, p. 11).

This concern has been raised in the past. The U.S. Government's General Accounting Office (now the Government Accountability Office) was fully aware that the domestic infant formula industry "is one of the most concentrated manufacturing industries in the country," with only three major producers since the 1970s (GAO, 1990, p. 21). In May 1990, the Senate Subcommittee on Antitrust, Monopolies, and Business Rights held a hearing on the pricing behavior of infant formula companies. The Federal Trade Commission also investigated potential anti-competitive practices in the industry. Charges of bid-rigging were brought against the three largest manufacturers (Baumslag & Michels, 1995, pp. 180-181; Oliveira, Prell, Smallwood, & Frazão, 2001, p. 33; also see Epstein, 1996; Fentiman, 2010, p. 54; Jovanovic, 1998). While these legal cases have been resolved, the potential for anti-competitive practices remains.

Third, the cost containment required under the procurement rules might save the government money, but it increases costs to consumers.

WIC compensates the retailers on the basis of their retail prices. Since WIC pays this amount without questioning it, the stores have a strong incentive to push their retail prices upward. Formula users who are not currently getting free formula from WIC have to pay the higher retail price for these brands. Data collected by the government show that where WIC clients are concentrated, retail prices for formula are higher (Betson & Smallwood, 2009; Oliveira et al., 2010).

The rebates from the manufacturers to WIC are close to 90 percent of the wholesale price, suggesting that the actual cost of production to the manufacturers is quite small. For name-brand formulas, the cost of the ingredients purchased by the manufacturer may be less than ten percent of the retail price (Dairy Exporter, 2011).

Obtaining WIC contracts is of high value to the manufacturers. A study by the U.S. Department of Agriculture reported:

> We find that the manufacturer holding the WIC contract brand accounted for the vast majority—84 percent—of all formula sold by the top three manufacturers. The impact of a switch in the manufacturer that holds the WIC contract was considerable. The market share of the manufacturer of the new WIC contract brand increased by an average 74 percentage points after winning the contract. Most of this increase was a direct effect of WIC recipients switching to the new WIC contract brand. However, manufacturers also realized a spillover effect from winning the WIC contract whereby sales of formula purchased outside of the program also increased (Oliveira et al., 2011, Abstract, p. i).

The manufacturers do not pay rebates for sales to families outside the WIC program. Similarly, they do not pay rebates for infant formula purchased by WIC clients who purchase their brand after their supply of free formula ends, at the child's first birthday.

The manufacturers of generic formula are unwilling to submit bids and give large rebates because their products do not command brand loyalty. As a leader in the Dutch baby food business observed, "People don't switch brands in baby food unless their baby is not well. Brand loyalty is passed on from mother to daughter; price is never an issue" (The Economist, 2006, para 6). The manufacturers bid for WIC contracts because the WIC program attracts many people to their brands.

The WIC program provides free formula only up to the child's first birthday. The manufacturers produce not only infant formula, but also "toddler milks" and other foods. The manufacturers view their involvement in the WIC program as way of attracting customers who will stay with them long after they stop getting free formula through WIC. The manufacturers are running a kind of addiction model, with the government distributing free samples for them.

The rebate-based cost containment program might appear to save the government money because it reduces the unit cost of the infant formula that is distributed through the program. However, as explained below, the program creates incentives that lead to WIC's distributing far more units than would be desirable in terms of infants' health. If healthcare costs were taken into account, it seems likely that overall this "cost containment" program actually increases costs to the government as well as to consumers.

The U.S. Department of Agriculture and its WIC program devote a great deal of effort to assessing the impact of the WIC formula distribution program on the economic interests of the manufacturers, Why don't they assess the program's impacts on the health of its clients?

Fourth, as mentioned above, overall the system may provide inappropriate incentives, resulting in more widespread use of infant formula than would be justified in terms of relevant health and cost considerations. According to Elizabeth Jensen and Miriam Labbok:

> These sole source rebates generate considerable resources for the program, and the acceptance of the rebates may serve to undermine the WIC program's efforts to promote breastfeeding in several ways. At the program policy level, the rebates may create a dependency on distributing formula so more families can be served from the rebate income. Furthermore, the use of the rebate resources may carry fewer federal mandates, allowing the possibility of more flexibility in their use. The fiscal incentive to purchase and provide formula is compounded further by the relative costs of the WIC food packages; the package for formula-fed infant/mother pairs is less expensive to WIC than the cost of food packages for exclusively breastfed infant/mother pairs (Jensen & Labbok, 2011, pp. 2-3).

About a quarter of WIC's caseload is based on funding from the rebates as shown in Figure 10.2:

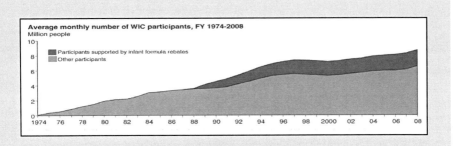

Figure 10.2. Average monthly number of WIC participants, FY 1974-2008 (million people)

Source: Oliveira V, Frazão E, Smallwood D. 2010. *Rising infant formula costs to the WIC Program: Recent trends in rebates and wholesale prices.* Washington, D.C.: U.S. Department of Agriculture. (http://www.ers.usda.gov/Publications/ERR93/)

Thus the rebate program helps WIC provide formula to more families.

Fifth, as pointed out earlier in the chapter on Additives, infant formula is sometimes regarded as a standardized commodity, and sometimes as a branded item with important differences among different versions of the product. WIC should assess the products offered by the manufacturers to determine whether the program, its clients, and taxpayers get good value from these contracts.

Sixth, the broad range of weaknesses in governmental regulation of infant formula together with WIC's large-scale provision of free infant formula suggests that there is, in effect, collusion between government and the infant formula industry. The cooperation between the government and the infant formula industry comes at the expense of the short and long term health of infants, and also results in increased costs for infant formula for people who are not getting free formula from WIC.

ISSUE 9. Procurement policies should be reviewed to ensure that they do not result in purchase of infant formula that is of questionable quality or overly costly to the government, program participants, or others outside the program.

11 Strengthening the Regulation of Infant Formula

Some people who were aware of the early global political struggles over the regulation of infant formula might have thought that with the adoption of the *International Code of Marketing of Breast-Milk Substitutes* (World Health Organization, 1981), the battle was won. However, there is much more to be done. Even a brief exploration of the websites of the International Baby Food Action Network and its affiliates, such as Baby Milk Action in England and INFACT in Canada, show that the struggle goes on. The persistence of the problems has been clearly demonstrated in the Philippines (Monbiot, 2007). This book has demonstrated that there are substantial problems in high-income as well as low-income countries.

The Code was a remarkable advance for its time, but it needs to be strengthened in several ways.

First, it needs to be made clear that the Code applies to all countries, not just low-income countries.

In the 1970s and 1980s, some people might have thought the problems with infant formula occurred in the low-income countries mainly because of their difficult living conditions. Attention should have been paid to the risks incurred everywhere (Akre, 2009, p. 5). It is now clear that infant formula results in worse health outcomes for infants in all populations, which means there is a problem with the product itself.

Some formula companies have tried to argue that the Marketing Code applies only to low-income countries, but it was intended from the outset to apply to all countries. Sami Shubber, the World Health Organization's Senior Legal Officer at the time of drafting the Code, is clear on this point:

> The International Code was adopted for the whole world and for all the membership of WHO, and there was no question of any distinction between developed and developing countries (Shubber, 1998, p. 44; also see Shubber, 2011).

The Code is an explicit part of the infant formula safety standards in many countries, including several high-income countries (IBFAN, 2009a, 2009b; NCT, 2010). Steps need to be taken to ensure the Code's full implementation in all countries.

Second, the Code needs to be updated to recognize that some governments promote the use of infant formula in a way that is contrary to the principles set out in the Code.

Currently, the Code focuses on manufacturers as the primary agencies to be regulated. Governments are viewed as the regulators. Governments certainly do have a role as regulators, but they need to be regulated as well. The Code should apply not only to manufacturers, but also to government agencies, hospitals, and others that have a role in child feeding.

Third, there is a need to clarify and strengthen the application of the Code in international trade and other international relations.

Infant formula is sold through international trade, much of it to low income countries. For example, the dairy industries in Australia and New Zealand export large quantities of infant formula to Asia and the Middle East. Fonterra supplies more than 65,000 tons of formula blends from its New Zealand and Australia manufacturing sites (Fonterra, 2010, p. 7). Some countries do not export infant formula, but export the milk solids, soy, and other ingredients of infant formula. Some export the technology and help other countries to set up their own manufacturing facilities. Often those factories are expected to purchase ingredients from the same country that provided the technology.

Under human rights principles, it is clear that exporters have some responsibilities if their products do harm in importing countries. The *International Code of Marketing of Breast-Milk Substitutes* does not say anything about international trade. However, *Codex Alimentarius* has a Code of Ethics for International Trade that says:

> National authorities should . . . make sure that the *international code of marketing of breast-milk substitutes* and relevant resolutions of the World Health Assembly (WHA) setting forth principles for the protection and promotion of breast-feeding be observed (Codex Alimentarius Commission, 2010, Section 4.4).

It is not clear whether any specific actions have been prompted by this guideline. The World Trade Organization (WTO) should clarify the application of the Code in international trade, and propose specific policies to implement it. For example, a policy could be adopted saying that countries that export infant formula should meet safety and effectiveness standards that are at least as stringent as those they impose on infant formula they produce or import.

Formally, Codex guidelines are advisory, but many countries now treat them as if they were binding. Some do this because the World Trade Organization uses them to guide its policies. In the WTO dispute settlement procedures, countries that follow Codex guidelines generally prevail over those that do not.

Regulations regarding the composition of foods and health claims associated with them vary a great deal across the world (Reis, 2011). Even if there were no international trade in infant formula, it would be useful to develop updated common global standards for infant formula, addressing not only its composition, but also its promotion and the claims that can be made for it.

Fourth, the Code is sometimes viewed as applying only to infant formula, so its applicability to other breast-milk substitutes needs to be clarified.

As explained by Nicholas Alipui of the United Nations Children's Fund:

> It is UNICEF's view that a follow-on formula is as much a breast-milk substitute as infant formula. Indeed, follow-on formulas did not exist when the *International Code of Marketing of Breast-milk Substitutes* was adopted in 1981, and were developed by the baby food industry to try and get around the prohibition on promotion in the Code. This led the World Health Assembly to adopt Resolution 39.28 in 1986 stating that "the practice being introduced in some countries of providing infants with specially formulated milks (so-called follow-up milks) is not necessary." Since, according to WHA [World Health Assembly], babies should be breastfed for two years or beyond, any milk product marketed for use before that age will replace breast-milk and must be considered a breast-milk substitute for the purposes of the Code (Alipui, 2011, para 2).

Fifth, the Code should be adapted and placed into the international human rights framework.

Several international human rights agreements relate to the nutrition of children, including:

- Universal Declaration of Human Rights
- International Covenant on Economic, Social and Cultural Rights

- Convention on the Elimination of All Forms of Discrimination Against Women
- Convention on the Rights of the Child

All current international human rights agreements can be accessed through the website of the Office of the High Commissioner for Human Rights, at http://www.ohchr.org.

Various human rights agreements have been used to clarify the human right to adequate food (Food and Agriculture Organization, 2005; Kent, 2005; United Nations Economic and Social Council, 1999). So far little attention has been given to the distinctive features of the nutrition of infants and young children. The role of international human rights law in relation to infant feeding was explored in my edited book on *Global Obligations for the Right to Food*, particularly in the chapters by Mike Brady of Baby Milk Action and Arun Gupta of the Breastfeeding Promotion Network of India (Kent, 2008).

The issues raised throughout this book could be addressed through a new Optional Protocol to the Convention on the Rights of the Child, and thus bring coherence to regulations relating to children's nutrition.

That Convention already has two Optional Protocols associated with it, one on the involvement of children in armed conflict, and another on the sale of children, child prostitution, and child pornography. Their forms could suggest a structure for a new Optional Protocol on Children's Nutrition, OPCN. The new Optional Protocol could present a set of widely agreed principles regarding the nutrition of children.

Working under the auspices of the United Nations General Assembly, the nations of the world could negotiate a draft OPCN. Drafts could be prepared by national governments working together with nongovernmental organizations. The drafters could draw from the many documents that already propose sound principles relating to children's nutrition, such as the World Health Organization's *Global*

Strategy for Infant and Young Child Feeding and the *International Code of Marketing of Breast-Milk Substitutes*. There are many other documents, now scattered, whose core ideas could be pulled together.

When a draft for the OPCN was ready, the General Assembly of the United Nations would vote on it. If a majority agreed, it would be adopted by the UN's General Assembly.

From that point forward, the executive branches of the national governments of the world would be invited to sign the OPCN, and then have their national legislatures or other appropriate bodies ratify it, in the normal procedure used to signify nations' agreements to international treaties.

Ratification would indicate the nation's acceptance of the OPCN and its commitment to conform its national laws to it. Following ratification, the broad principles stated in the OPCN would be given concrete form through the adoption of appropriate national laws. The ratification would signify the nation's willingness to be held accountable with regard to the principles stated in the OPCN, and the new national laws would be the means by which its leaders would act on its commitment.

The OPCN would not replace international bodies such as UNICEF and the Codex Alimentarius Commission, nor would it replace national regulatory agencies such as the Food and Drug Administration in the U.S. The OPCN would help to harmonize the work of all participating countries at the national level. It would be the apex document, setting out important principles relating to the nutrition of infants and young children.

One of the basic principles would be that infants and young children have a right to foods that are both safe and nutritionally adequate. The concepts would be defined at the global level, but implemented concretely at the national level. The widely accepted principles would be implemented through national legislation.

The drafters of the OPCN would have to accommodate diversity and recognize the important differences in cultural approaches to raising children in different places (DeLoache & Gottlieb, 2000). As a global document, it would focus mainly on widely accepted principles, and leave the details of implementation to be worked out in different countries according to their particular circumstances.

National regulatory and operational bodies, while functioning independently, would be free to obtain guidance from relevant global agencies such as the United Nations Children's Fund, the Food and Agriculture Organization of the United Nations, and the World Health Organization.

In time, another document could be prepared to suggest concrete ways in which national governments could implement the principles of the OPCN, comparable to the *Voluntary Guidelines to Support the Progressive Realization of the Right to Adequate Food in the Context of National Food Security* (Food and Agriculture Organization, 2005).

This approach would place children's nutrition decisively into the human rights framework. Like other forms of international law, it would not result in immediate compliance, but it would establish clear and widely agreed standards, and it would support the preparation of strong law at the national level. A new Optional Protocol on Children's Nutrition, linked to the Convention on the Rights of the Child, would help to establish coherent regulations for ensuring that infants and young children everywhere are well nourished.

Until that can be accomplished, all levels of governance, including sub-national, national, and global levels, should do what they can to strengthen regulations relating to infant and young child nutrition.

ISSUE 10.	Regulations governing the ways in which infant formula is produced, marketed, and used should be strengthened at every level.

12 | Future Work

Direct violence is the type encountered in muggings, murders, and armed conflicts. There is also such a thing as indirect or structural violence. Structural violence is harm imposed by some people on others indirectly through the social system, as they pursue their own preferences. Structural violence can be small-scale and quiet. For example, if many rich people begin moving into a community, they will drive up housing costs, harming some of the people who had already lived there. The harms are real, even if they are not inflicted deliberately.

With direct violence, there is a specific event, an identifiable victim, and an identifiable perpetrator. In contrast, structural violence is not visible in specific events. Its effects are observable at the societal level as systematic shortfalls in the quality of life of certain groups of people. In direct violence, there is physical damage to the human body occurring in a distinct event, and victims and perpetrators can be identified. In structural violence, however, people suffer harm indirectly, often through a slow and steady process, with no clearly identifiable perpetrators. Structural violence cannot be photographed. It is revealed only through its patterned effects. Most victims of homelessness or chronic malnutrition, for example, are victims of structural violence.

The systematic structural violence against children is not directly visible, but its effects show up in the record of child mortality worldwide (Kent,

1991, 2011). While there has been good progress in reducing child mortality, there are still more than eight million children that die before their fifth birthdays every year.

Many factors contribute to this high level of mortality. Standard infant formula used in the general population increases the child mortality in high-income countries as well as in low-income countries. It may be that special infant formulas sometimes save the lives of infants with unusual needs, but overall there are greater harms that result from the widespread use of standard infant formula.

This book has demonstrated systematic failures in the system of regulation for infant formula:

- Regulations have been based on the assumption that any formula for which the basic ingredients match up with a list of ingredients is *safe*, despite abundant evidence that the assumption is not correct.

- Regulations have been based on the assumption that any formula for which the basic ingredients match up with a list of ingredients is *nutritionally adequate*, despite abundant evidence that the assumption is not correct.

- Regulations are not based on systematic assessment of the effectiveness of each variety of infant formula in ensuring the healthy development of infants.

- Various additives to infant formula are assumed to be safe and effective, despite evidence to the contrary.

- Regulations are based on the assumption that formula will be used in an optimal way, despite the abundant evidence that it is not.

- The issue of water quality is ignored.

- Little effort has been made to provide clear information on risks, in a suitable form, to allow parents and policymakers to make well informed choices.

- There is no clear system in place to protect infants from outdated and recalled infant formula.

- Improper marketing of infant formula continues despite the clear guidelines in the *International Code of Marketing of Breast-Milk Substitutes*.

- Neither manufacturers nor governments undertake fair studies of the health and economic impacts of using infant formula to the extent they are needed to protect children's health.

- Some government agencies provide infant formula at no cost, promoting its use, and thus undermine their campaigns to support breastfeeding.

The ten issues identified in the preceding chapters are listed in the Appendix, together with this list of examples of major failures.

If the health and development of children were to become the primary concern of the regulators, the precautionary principle would lead them to make assumptions exactly the opposite of the ones they have been making. In that new world, no one would even suggest that infant formula made from genetically modified soy is so obviously safe as to not require testing. Serious testing would include assessment of long-term as well as short-term effects.

The individual weaknesses in the system for regulating infant formula, viewed in isolation, might be regarded as simple flaws in management, but the overview offered here reveals a glaring pattern: *Current regulations for infant formula systematically and regularly favor the interests of the manufacturers of infant formula over the interests of infants, exposing infants everywhere to excessive risks to their health.*

The use of infant formula regularly leads to worse health outcomes than would be obtained with breastfeeding. This cannot be viewed as a simple, transitory mistake. Alarms have been raised for decades, and they have not been addressed with the seriousness they require. The system of regulation needs to be thoroughly overhauled, at every level, from global to local, to provide children with the protection they need and deserve.

Not only regulatory agencies, but also operational agencies of national and sub-national governments could take a more active role in shaping the policies under which they operate. An Optional Protocol on Children's Nutrition, linked to the United Nations Convention on the Rights of the Child, could set out widely agreed fundamental principles relating to child nutrition.

New guidelines could be developed at every level, building on those already provided in documents such as the *International Code of Marketing of Breast-Milk Substitutes*, the Baby Friendly Hospital Initiative, and the World Health Organization and UNICEF's guidance for infant and young child feeding.

The quickest and most practical approach to strengthening regulations would be for all agencies involved in the nutrition of infants and young children to recognize their responsibilities for ensuring that children are well nourished. There is no good reason to accept the weaknesses of the present system. All agencies with a role in child feeding should insist on a system of regulation that consistently serves the best interests not of corporations, but of children.

References

Academy of Breastfeeding Medicine. (2011). Educational objectives and skills for the physician with respect to breastfeeding. *Breastfeeding Medicine, 6,* 2. Retrieved on August 16, 2011, from http://www.bfmed.org/Media/Files/Documents/pdf/Statements/ABM Statement bfm.2011.9994.pdf

Agricultural Research Service. (2004, January). Study examines long-term health effects of soy infant formula. *Agricultural Research,* 52(2), 8-10. Retrieved on August 16, 2011, from http://www.ars.usda.gov/is/AR/archive/jan04/soy0104.pdf

Akre, J. (2006). *The problem with breastfeeding: A personal reflection.* Amarillo, Texas: Hale Publishing.

Akre, J. (2009). From grand design to change on the ground: Going to scale with a global feeding strategy. In F. Dykes & V. Hall-Moran (Eds.), *Infant and young child feeding.* New York: Wiley-Blackwell. Retrieved on August 16, 2011, from http://www.wiley.com/WileyCDA/WileyTitle/productCd-1405187212.html

Akre, J. E., Gribble, K.D., & Minchin, M. (2011). Milk sharing: From private practice to public pursuit. *International Breastfeeding Journal, 6*(8). Retrieved on August 16, 2011, from http://www.internationalbreastfeedingjournal.com/content/6/1/8/abstract

Alipui, N. (2011). UNICEF expresses its support for the Resolution opposing the health claim. *Babymilk Action.* Retrieved on August 16, 2011, from http://info.babymilkaction.org/news/policyblog/unicefDHA

American Academy of Pediatrics. (1998). Soy protein-based formulas: recommendations for use in infant feeding. *Pediatrics, 101*(1), 148-153. Retrieved on August 16, 2011, from http://aappolicy.aappublications.org/cgi/reprint/pediatrics;101/1/148.pdf

American Academy of Pediatrics. (2005). Breastfeeding and the use of human milk. *Pediatrics, 115*(2), 496-506. Retrieved on August 22, 2011, from http://pediatrics.aappublications.org/content/115/2/496.full.pdf+html

American Dietetic Association. (2001). Position of the American Dietetic Association: Breaking the barriers to breastfeeding. *Journal of the American Dietetic Association, 101*(10), 1213-1220.

Armenian Forum. (1998). *After infant formula debacle, Armenia goes back to basics.* Retrieved on August 16, 2011, from http://www.gomidas.org/forum/af2milk.htm

Australia. (2011, March). *Regulatory impact statement: Policy guideline for the regulation of infant formula products.* Retrieved on August 16, 2011, from http://ris.finance.gov.au/files/2011/05/Infant_Formula_Products_RIS.pdf

Baby Center. (2011). *Are generic or store-brand formulas less nutritious than brand-name formulas?* Retrieved on August 16, 2011, from http://www.babycenter.com/404_are-generic-or-store-brand-formulas-less-nutritious-than-bra_1334547.bc

Baby-Friendly USA, Inc. (2011). *Implementing the UNICEF/WHO Baby Friendly Hospital Initiative in the U.S.* Retrieved on August 16, 2011, from http://www.babyfriendlyusa.org/

Baby Milk Action. (2011a, March). *STOP PRESS: EU MEPs oppose follow-on milk claim.* Retrieved August 16, 2011, from http://info.babymilkaction.org/news/policyblog/dhabriefing

Baby Milk Action. (2011b, March). *Companies stop using DHA claims in the USA. California WIC write to MEPs.* Retrieved August 16, 2010, from http://info.babymilkaction.org/news/policyblog/DHAusa

Baby Milk Action. (2011c, April). *European Parliament votes to block DHA health claim – but not by a large enough majority to guarantee action by the Commission.* Retrieved August 16, 2010, from http://info.babymilkaction.org/pressrelease/pressrelease06apr11

Badger, T.M., Gilchrist, J.M., Pivik, R.T., Andres, A., Shankar, K., Chen, J.R., & Ronis, M.J. (2009). The health implications of soy infant formula. *American Journal of Clinical Nutrition, 89*(5 suppl.), 1668S-1672S. Retrieved on August 16, 2011, from http://www.ajcn.org/content/89/5/1668S.full

Baker, R.D. (2002). Commentary: Infant formula safety. *Pediatrics, 110*(4), 833-835. Retrieved on August 16, 2011, from http://pediatrics.aappublications.org/cgi/content/full/110/4/833

Bardelline, J. (2011a, March). China, Malaysia become latest nations to ban BPA. *Greener Design.* Retrieved August 16, 2011, from http://www.greenbiz.com/news/2011/03/14/china-malaysia-latest-nations-ban-bpa

Bardelline, J. (2011b, January). BPA bans, chemical reform laws in the works in 30 states. *Greener Design.* Retrieved August 16, 2011, from http://www.greenbiz.com/news/2011/01/18/bpa-bans-chemical-reform-laws-works-30-states

Barnett, A. (2004, November). They hailed it as a wonderfood: Soya not only destroys forests and small farmers—it can also be bad for your health. *The Observer*. Retrieved August 16, 2011, from http://observer.guardian.co.uk/foodmonthly/story/0,9950,1342291,00.html

Bartick, M. & Reinhold, A. (2010). The burden of suboptimal breastfeeding in the United States: A pediatric cost analysis. *Pediatrics, 125*(5), e1048-56. Retrieved August 23, 2011, from http://pediatrics.aappublications.org/content/125/5/e1048.full.pdf

Baumslag, N. & Michels, D.L. (1995). *Milk, money, and madness: The culture and politics of breastfeeding*. Westport, Connecticut: Bergin & Garvey.

Baumslag, N. (ed.). (2006). *Mother & child health—Common sense, creativity and care. Selected works of Dr. Cicely D. Williams, primary health care pioneer*. Penang, Malaysia: World Alliance for Breastfeeding Action.

BDNews.com. (2011, May). *Donors attacked for going commercial to tackle malnutrition*. Retrieved on August 16, 2011, from http://bdnews24.com/details.php?id=196688&cid=13

Betson, D. & Smallwood, D. (2009, January). *Impact of the WIC Program on the infant formula market*. Washington, D.C.: U.S. Department of Agriculture. Report No. 51. Retrieved August 16, 2011, from http://ddr.nal.usda.gov/dspace/handle/10113/32816

Bhatia, J., Greer, F., American Academy of Pediatrics Committee on Nutrition. (2008). Use of soy protein-based formulas in infant feeding. *Pediatrics, 121*(5), 1062-1068. Retrieved on August 16, 2011, from http://pediatrics.aappublications.org/cgi/content/abstract/121/5/1062

Birch, L.L., Parker, L., & Burns, A. (Eds.). (2011, June). *Early childhood obesity prevention policies*. Washington, D.C.: Institute of Medicine. Retrieved on August 16, 2011, from http://www.iom.edu/Reports/2011/Early-Childhood-Obesity-Prevention-Policies.aspx

British Dietetic Association. (2003). Paediatric group position statement on the use of soya protein for infants. *Journal of Family Health Care, 13*(4), 93. Retrieved on August 16, 2011, from http://www.ncbi.nlm.nih.gov/entrez/query.fcgi?cmd=Retrieve&db=PubMed&list_uids=14528647&dopt=Abstract

Burros, M. (1995, September). Eating Well; F.D.A. Target: Baby Formula. *New York Times*. Retrieved August 16, 2011, from http://www.nytimes.com/1995/09/06/garden/eating-well-fda-target-baby-formula.html

Burrows, V.K. (2007). *CRS Report for Congress. The FDA's authority to recall products*. Washington, D.C.: Congressional Research Service. Retrieved on August 16, 2011, from http://opencrs.com/document/RL34167/2007-09-11/download/1005/

Butte, N.F., Lopez-Alarcon, M.G., & Garza, C. (2002). *Nutrient adequacy of exclusive breastfeeding for the term infant during the first six months of life.* Geneva, Switzerland: World Health Organization. Retrieved on August 16, 2011, from http://www.who.int/entity/nutrition/publications/infantfeeding/9241562110/en/

California WIC Association. (2010). *Concerns about infant formula marketing and additives.* Retrieved August 16, 2011, from http://www.calwic.org/storage/documents/federal/2010/formulabrief.pdf

Chen, A., & Rogan, W.J. (2004). Breastfeeding and the risk of postneonatal death in the United States. *Pediatrics, 113*(5), 435-439.

Codex Alimentarius Commission. (1976). *Statement on infant feeding, CAC/MISC-2-1976.* Retrieved on August 16, 2011, from http://www.codexalimentarius.net/download/standards/301/CXA_002e.pdf

Codex Alimentarius Commission. (1981). *Standard for infant formula and formulas for special medical purposes intended for infants.* CODEX STAN 72-108. Retrieved August 16, 2011, from http://www.codexalimentarius.net/download/standards/288/CXS_072e.pdf

Codex Alimentarius Commission. (1989). *Codex general guidelines for the utilization of vegetable protein products (VPP) in foods.* CAC/GL 4-1989. Retrieved August 16, 2011, from http://www.codexalimentarius.net/download/standards/326/CXG_004e.pdf

Codex Alimentarius Commission. (2007). *Standard for infant formula and formulas for special medical purposes intended for infants.* CODEX STAN 72-108. [Formerly CAC/RS 72-1972. Adopted as a world-wide Standard 1981. Amended 1983, 1985, 1987. Revision 2007]. Retrieved on August 16, 2011, from http://www.codexalimentarius.net/download/standards/288/CXS_072e.pdf

Codex Alimentarius Commission. (2008). *Code of hygienic practice for powdered formulae for infants and young children.* CAC/RCP 66 – 2008. Retrieved on August 16, 2011, from http://www.codexalimentarius.net/download/standards/11026/CXP_066e.pdf

Codex Alimentarius Commission. (2010). *Code of ethics for international trade in food including concessional and food aid transactions.* CAC/RCP 20-1979. [Adopted in 1979. Revised in 1985 and 2010]. Retrieved August 16, 2011, from http://www.codexalimentarius.net/download/standards/1/CXP_020e.pdf

Codex Alimentarius Commission. (2011). FAO/WHO food standards - codex alimentarius. Retrieved on August 16, 2011, from http://www.codexalimentarius.net/web/index_en.jsp

Collier, R. (2011). Squabble over risks of probiotics infant formula. *CMAJ (Canadian Medical Association Journal), 181*(3-4), E46-E47. Retrieved on August 16, 2011, from http://www.cmaj.ca/content/181/3-4/E46.full.pdf+html

Crawley, H. & Westland, S. (2011). *Infant milks in the UK.* Abbots Langley, United Kingdom: Caroline Walker Trust. Retrieved on August 16, 2011, from http://www.cwt.org.uk/pdfs/infantsmilk_web.pdf

Crienglish.com. (2011, June). *Infant formula to be inspected monthly.* Retrieved on August 16, 2011, from http://english.cri. cn/6909/2011/06/08/2681s641719.htm

CTV News. (2003, January). *Heinz goes green, guarantees baby food GMO-free.* Retrieved on August 16, 2011, from http://www.ctv.ca/servlet/ArticleNews/story/CTVNews/1043968381082_39377581/

Dairy Exporter. (2011). *Infant formula – A 'superstar' that's still expanding.* New Zealand Dairy Exporter. Retrieved on August 16, 2011, from http://www.dairyexporter.co.nz/article/36353.html

Daniel, K. 2005. *The Whole Soy Story: The Dark Side of America's Favorite Health Food.* Winona Lake, Indiana: New Trends Publishing. Also see website at http://blog.wholesoystory.com/

de la Torre, V.M. (2011, March). *Stop this marketing ploy on baby milk.* Group of the Progressive Alliance of Socialists & Democrats in the European Parliament. Retrieved on August 16, 2011, from http://www.socialistgroup.eu/gpes/public/detail.htm?id=135499&request_locale=EN&section=NER&category=NEWS

DeLoache, J. & Gottlieb, A. (2000). *A world of babies: Imagined childcare guides for seven societies.* Cambridge, United Kingdom: Cambridge University Press.

Democracy Now. (2005, June). *Milk money: How corporate interests shaped government health policy for women.* Retrieved on August 16, 2011, from http://www.democracynow.org/2005/6/23/milk_money_how_corporate_interests_shaped

De Onis, M., Garza, C., Victora, C.G., Bhan, M.K., & Norum, K.R. (2004). The WHO Multicentre Growth Reference Study (MGRS): Rationale, planning, and implementation. *Food and Nutrition Bulletin,* 25, No. 1. Retrieved on August 16, 2011, from http://www.who.int/childgrowth/mgrs/fnu/en/index.html

Devaney, B., & Schrim, A. (1993). *Infant mortality among Medicaid newborns in 5 states: The effects of prenatal WIC participation.* Princeton, New Jersey: Mathematica Policy Research.

DiMesio, R. (2008, December). Expired food not illegal in Oregon. OregonLive. com. Retrieved on August 16, 2011, from http://blog.oregonlive.com/complaintdesk/2008/12/expired_food_not_illegal_in_or.html

Dorfman, L. & Gehler, H. (2010). *Talking about breastfeeding: Why the health argument isn't enough.* Berkeley, California: Berkeley Media Studies Group. Retrieved on August 16, 2011, from http://www.bmsg.org/pdfs/BMSG_Issue_18.pdf

Dugger, C.W. (2005, August). Where a cuddle with your baby requires a bribe. *New York Times.* Retrieved on August 16, 2011, from http://www.nytimes.com/2005/08/30/international/asia/30bangalore.html

Earthweek. (2011, March). *Human-like milk from cows developed in China.* Retrieved on August 16, 2011, from http://www.earthweek.com/2011/ew110325/ew110325e.html

EFSA Panel on Dietetic Projects, Nutrition and Allergies. (2009). DHA and ARA and visual development - Scientific substantiation of a health claim related to docosahexaenoic acid (DHA) and arachidonic acid (ARA) and visual development pursuant to Article14 of Regulation (EC) No 1924/2006[1]. *EFSA Journal*. February 13. Retrieved on August 23, 2011, from http://www.efsa.europa.eu/en/efsajournal/pub/941.htm

Emergency Nutrition Network. (2011, April). *Draft guidance on marketing regulation of RUSF*. Retrieved on August 16, 2011, from http://www.ennonline.net/resources/768

Engle, P.L., Menon, P., & Haddad, L. 1997. *Care and nutrition: Concepts and measurement*. Washington, D.C.: International Food Policy Research Institute. Retrieved on August 16, 2011, from http://www.ifpri.org/sites/default/files/publications/oc33.pdf

Epstein, L. (1996). Women and children last: Anti-competitive practices in the infant formula industry. *American University Journal of Gender & the Law, 5*(1).

Esterik, P.V. (2002). *Risks, rights and regulation: Communicating about risks and infant feeding*. Penang, Malaysia: World Alliance for Breastfeeding Action. Retrieved on August 16, 2011, from http://www.waba.org.my/whatwedo/environment/penny.htm

Euromonitor International. (2010, November). *Baby food in Israel*. Retrieved on August 16, 2011, from http://www.euromonitor.com/baby-food-in-israel/report

Euromonitor International. (2011, January). *Baby food in the US. Trends*. Retrieved on August 16, 2011, from http://www.euromonitor.com/baby-food-in-the-us/report

EUR-Lex, (2011). Commission Directive 2006/141/EC of 22 December 2006 on infant formulae and follow-on formulae and amending Directive 1999/21/EC (1). *Eur-Lex, 49*. Retrieved on August 16, 2011, from http://eur-lex.europa.eu/JOHtml.do?uri=OJ:L:2006:401:SOM:EN:HTML

European Parliament. (2011, April). *DHA in baby food: European Parliament approves health claim*. Retrieved on August 16, 2011, from http://www.europarl.europa.eu/en/pressroom/content/20110406IPR17110/html/DHA-in-baby-food-European-Parliament-approves-health-claim

European Union Register of nutrition and health claims made on food – Authorized health claims (2011). Article 14(1)(b) health claims referring to children's development and health. Retrieved on August 25, 2011, from http://ec.europa.eu/food/food/labellingnutrition/claims/community_register/authorised_health_claims_en.htm

FDA scientists questions soy safety - but where is GM testing? (2004). Retrieved on August 16, 2011, from http://www.netlink.de/gen/Zeitung/2000/000609.html

Fentiman, L.C. (2010). Marketing mothers' milk: The commodification of breastfeeding and the new markets for breast milk and infant formula. *Nevada Law Journal* (10)1. Retrieved on August 16, 2011, from http://scholars.law.unlv.edu/nlj/vol10/iss1/3/

Fewtrell, M.S. (2004). The long-term benefits of having been breastfed. *Current Pediatrics, 14,* 97-103.

Field, M. (2011, May). "Kiwi" firms are made in China. *Business Day.* Retrieved on August 16, 2011, from http://www.stuff.co.nz/business/5101783/Kiwi-firms-are-made-in-China

Fomon, S.J. (2004). Assessment of growth of formula-fed infants: Evolutionary considerations. *Pediatrics, 113*(2), 389-393. Retrieved on August 16, 2011, from http://pediatrics.aappublications.org/cgi/content/full/113/2/389

Fonterra. (2010). *About Fonterra.* Auckland, New Zealand: Fonterra Co-operative Group Limited. Retrieved August 16, 2011, from http://www.fonterra.com/wps/wcm/connect/f4b20680449b4a5b86c697a9c2d85acf/About+Fonterra+-+Nov+2010c.pdf?MOD=AJPERES&CACHEID=f4b20680449b4a5b86c697a9c2d85acf

Food and Agriculture Organization of the United Nations. (2005). *Voluntary guidelines to support the progressive realization of the right to adequate food in the context of national food security.* Rome: FAO. Retrieved on August 16, 2011, from http://www.fao.org/docrep/meeting/009/y9825e/y9825e00.htm

GAO. (1990, September). *Infant formula: Cost containment and competition in the WIC program.* Washington, D.C.: U.S. General Accounting Office. GAO/HRD-90-122. Retrieved on August 16, 2011, from http://archive.gao.gov/d23t8/142337.pdf

GAO. (1992, April). *Early intervention: Federal investments like WIC can produce savings.* Washington, D.C.: U. S. General Accounting Office. GAO/HRD-92-18. Retrieved on August 16, 2011, from http://archive.gao.gov/d32t10/146514.pdf

Garza, C., & de Onis, M. (1999). A new international growth reference for young children. *American Journal of Clinical Nutrition, 70*(1), 169S-172S. Retrieved on August 16, 2011, from http://www.ajcn.org/cgi/content/full/70/1/169S?maxtoshow=&HITS=10&hits=10&RESULTFORMA

Goldberg, G.R., Prentice, A., Prentice, A., Filteau, S., Simondon, K. (2009). *Breast-feeding: Early influences on later health.* (Advances in Experimental Medicine and Biology, Vol. 639). New York: Springer Publishers.

Good Food. (2011, March). Genetically modified cows produce "human" milk. Retrieved on August 16, 2011, from http://www.good.is/post/genetically-modified-cows-produce-human-milk/

Gribble, K.D., McGrath, M., MacLaine, A., & Lhotska, L. (2011). Supporting breastfeeding in emergencies: protecting women's reproductive rights and maternal and infant health. *Disasters.* doi:10.1111/j.1467-7717.2011.01239.x

Hale, T.W. (2010). *Medications and mother's milk.* Amarillo, Texas: Hale Publishing.

Heikkilä, K., Sacker, A., Yvonne Kelly, Y., Renfrew, M.J., & Quigley, M.A. (2011). Breast feeding and child behaviour in the Millennium Cohort Study. *Archives of Disease in Childhood.* 96:635-642. doi:10.1136/adc.2010.201970.

Heinig, J.M., Goldbronn, J., & Bañuelos, J. (2010). *Limited effectiveness of long-chain polyunsaturated fatty acids in infant formula: Is universal use of these supplements justified?* Sacramento, California: California WIC Association and UC Davis Human Lactation Center. Retrieved on August 16, 2011, from http://info.babymilkaction.org/sites/info.babymilkaction.org/files/LCPF%20study%20FINAL_0.pdf

Hester, T. (2010, October). *Wal-Mart agrees to pay state $775,000 for selling expired infant formula and over-the-counter drugs.* Retrieved on August 16, 2011, from http://www.newjerseynewsroom.com/healthquest/wal-mart-agrees-to-pay-state-775000-for-selling-expired-infant-formula-and-over-the-counter-drugs

Horwood, L. J., & Fergusson, D.M. (1998). Breastfeeding and later cognitive and academic outcome. *Pediatrics, 101*(1), e9. Retrieved on August 16, 2011, from http://pediatrics.aappublications.org/cgi/content/full/101/1/e9

IBFAN. (2009a). *European countries downgraded.* Retrieved on August 16, 2010, from http://www.ibfan.org/regional_news-europe.html

IBFAN. (2009b). *State of the code by country.* Retrieved on August 16, 2010, from http://www.ibfan.org/code_watch-reports.html

IBFAN. (2010). *STOP PRESS: Global concern is increasing rapidly over the adverse effects of low doses of the chemical Bisphenol A, BPA, on the development of the brain and the nervous system in infants and young children.* Retrieved on August 16, 2011, from http://www.ibfan.org/parents_20100413.html.

IBFAN. (2011). *International Baby Food Action Network.* Retrieved on August 16, 2011, from http://www.ibfan.org/

INFACT Canada. (1997). Fools gold: Recommendation - Strong buy. *Spring 1997 Newsletter.* Breastfeeding Protection: Code Watch. Retrieved on August 16, 2011, from http://www.infactcanada.ca/codewach.htm

INFACT Canada. (2002). *Fourteen risks of formula feeding: A brief annotated bibliography by the Breastfeeding Action Group in Corner Brook, Newfoundland.* Toronto: INFACT Canada. Retrieved on August 16, 2011, from http://www.infactcanada.ca/pdf/14-Risks-Small.pdf

Infant Formula Council. (2010). *Positive health contributions of infant formula.* Retrieved on August 16, 2011, from http://www.infantformula.org/newsroom/press-releases-and-statements/positive-health-contributions-infant-formula

Infant Formula Council. (2011). *What nutrients are present in infant formula and why are they included?* Retrieved on August 16, 2011, from http://www.infantformula.org/faqs

Infant Nutrition Council. (2011). *Infant formula information*. Retrieved on August 16, 2011, from http://infantnutritioncouncil.com/formula-information/

Institute of Medicine. Committee on the Evaluation of the Addition of Ingredients New to Infant Formula. (2004). *Infant formula: Evaluating the safety of new ingredients*. Washington, D.C.: National Academies Press. Retrieved on August 16, 2011, from http://www.nap.edu/openbook. php?isbn=0309091500

Institute of Medicine. (2005). *WIC food packages: Time for a change*. Washington, D.C.: National Academies Press. Retrieved on August 16, 2011, from http:// www.iom.edu/Reports/2005/WIC-Food-Packages-Time-for-a-Change.aspx

Isanaka, S., Nombela, N., Djibo, A., Poupard, M., Van Beckhoven, D., Gaboulaud, V., et al. (2009). Effect of preventive supplementation with ready-to-use therapeutic food on the nutritional status, mortality, and morbidity of children aged 6 to 60 months in Niger. A cluster randomized trial. *Journal American Medical Association, 301*(3), 277-285. Retrieved on August 16, 2011, from http://jama.ama-assn.org/content/301/3/277.full. pdf+html?sid=c4867441-c117-4662-acce-c8c110ae2b86

Jensen, E.., & Labbok, M. (2011). Unintended consequences of the WIC formula rebate program on infant feeding outcomes: Will the new food packages be enough? *Breastfeeding Medicine, 6*(3), 145-149. Retrieved on August 16, 2011, from http://www.sph.unc.edu/images/stories/centers_institutes/CIYCFC/ Documents/jensen_e_and_labbok_m,_wic_formula_rebate.pdf

Johnson, L.N. (2011, June). Drop-side cribs ban takes effect, users have time to comply. *International Business Times*. Retrieved on August 16, 2011, from http://www.ibtimes.com/articles/170690/20110628/aap-drop-side-cpsc-consumer-national-institute-of-child-health-and-human-development-ban-crib-baby-s.htm

Jovanovic, D. (1998). *Anticompetitive Issues in the Infant Formula Industry*. Master's Thesis. Youngstown, Ohio: Youngstown State University. Retrieved on August 16, 2011, from http://etd.ohiolink.edu/view.cgi/Jovanovic%20 Dusan.pdf?ysu997197215

Keller and Heckman LLP. (2009, July). *Connecticut bans BPA in all infant formula and baby food containers*. Washington, D.C. Retrieved on August 16, 2011, from http://www.packaginglaw.com/2904_.shtml

Kennell, J.H., & Klaus, M.H. (1998). Bonding: Recent observations that alter perinatal care. *Pediatrics in Review, 19*(1), 4-12.

Kent, G. (1991). *The politics of children's survival*. New York: Praeger Publishers.

Kent, G. (2005). *Freedom from want: The human right to adequate food*. Washington, D.C.: Georgetown University Press. Retrieved on August 16, 2011, from http://press.georgetown.edu/sites/default/files/978-1-58901-055-0%20 w%20CC%20license.pdf

Kent, G. (2006). WIC's promotion of infant formula in the United States. *International Breastfeeding Journal, 1*, 8. Retrieved on August 16, 2011, from http://www.internationalbreastfeedingjournal.com/content/1/1/8

Kent, G. (Ed.). (2008). *Global obligations for the right to food.* New York: Rowman & Littlefield.

Kent, G. (2011). *Ending hunger worldwide.* Boulder, Colorado: Paradigm Publishers.

Koletzko, B. & Shamir, R. (2006). Editorial: Standards for infant formula milk: Commercial interests may be the strongest driver of what goes into formula milk. *British Medical Journal,* 16 March. Retrieved on August 16, 2011, from http://www.bmj.com/content/332/7542/621.extract

Kristof, N. (2011, June). The breast milk cure. *New York Times.* Retrieved on August 16, 2011, from http://www.nytimes.com/2011/06/23/opinion/23kristof.html?_r=1&emc=eta1

Labbok, M., Clark, D., & Goldman, A. (2004). Breastfeeding: Maintaining an irreplaceable immunological resource. *Nature Reviews: Immunology, 4,* 565-572.

Lane, Y. (2010, September). GM protestors want baby formula out. *International Business Times.* Retrieved on August 16, 2011, from http://au.ibtimes.com/articles/65765/20100927/gm-protesters-want-baby-formula-out.htm

Latham, M. (1997). *Human nutrition in the developing world.* Rome: Food and Agriculture Organization of the United Nations.

Latham, M., Jonsson, U., Sterken, E., & Kent, G. 2011. RUTF stuff. Can the children be saved with fortified peanut paste? *World Nutrition,* 2(2), 62-85. Retrieved on August 16, 2011, from http://www.wphna.org/2011_feb_wn3_comm_RUTF.htm

Lawrence, R.A., & Lawrence, R. 2011. *Breastfeeding: A guide for the medical profession,* (7th ed.). Maryland Heights, Missouri: Elsevier Mosby.

Leiss, W., & Powell, D. (2004). *Mad cows and mother's milk: The perils of poor risk communication.* Montreal and Kingston, Canada: McGill-Queen's University Press.

León-Cava, N., Lutter, C., Ross, J., & Martin, L. (2002). *Quantifying the benefits of breastfeeding: A summary of the evidence.* Washington, D.C.: Pan American Health Organization. Retrieved on August 16, 2011, from http://www.paho.org/English/AD/FCH/BOB-Main.htm

Lönnerdal, B. 2002. Expression of human milk proteins in plants. *Journal of the American College of Nutrition, 21*(3), 218S-2221S. Retrieved on August 16, 2011, from http://www.jacn.org/cgi/reprint/21/suppl_3/218S

Lönnerdal, B., & Kelleher, S.L. (2007, December). Iron metabolism in infants and children. *Food and Nutrition Bulletin, 28*(3 Supply), S491-499.

Lucas, A., Stafford, M., Morley, R., Abbott, R., Stephenson, T., MacFadyen, U., et al. (1999). Efficacy and safety of long-chain polyunsaturated fatty acid supplementation of infant-formula milk: a randomised trial. *Lancet, 354*(9194), 1948-1954. Retrieved on August 16, 2011, from http://www.thelancet.com/search/results?fieldName=Authors&searchTerm=Mai+Stafford

Lunder, S., & Houlihan, J. (2007). EWG's guide to infant formula and baby bottles. *Environmental Working Group.* Retrieved on August 16, 2011, from http://www.ewg.org/reports/infantformula

Martek. (2009a). Martek to be the sole-source supplier of DHA and ARA for Prodigy brand infant formula products in China. Columbia, Maryland: Market Biosciences Corporation. Retrieved on August 16, 2011, from http://newsroom.martek.com/index.php?s=5256&item=3314

Martek. (2009b). Martek to be the sole source supplier of DHA and ARA for infant formulas produced by Grupo Ricap. Columbia, Maryland: Martek Biosciences. Retrieved on August 16, 2011, from http://newsroom.martek.com/index.php?s=5256&item=3300

Martek. (2009c). *Martek signs sole-source supply agreement with Fonterra.* Columbia, Maryland: Martek Biosciences Corporation. Retrieved on August 16, 2011, from http://investors.martek.com/releasedetail.cfm?releaseid=429369

Martek. (2011). *The importance of DHA and ARA in infant development.* Martek Biosciences Corporation. Retrieved on August 16, 2011, from http://www.martek.com/Healthcare-Professionals/Clinical-Research/Infant-Development/tabid/135/Default.aspx

Martin, A. (2011, January). Consumer agency tightens scrutiny of baby sleep products. *New York Times.* Retrieved on August 16, 2011, from http://www.nytimes.com/2011/02/01/business/01safety.html?ref=andrewmartin

Martyn, T. (2003). Artificial baby milks: How safe is soya? *Midwives, 6*(5), 212-215. Retrieved on August 31, 2011, from http://www.babymilkaction.org/pdfs/tessaysoya03.pdf

McNiel, M., Labbok, M., & Abrahams, S.W. 2010. What are the risks associated with formula feeding? A re-analysis and review. *Birth, 37*(1), 50-58. Retrieved on August 16, 2011, from http://onlinelibrary.wiley.com/doi/10.1111/j.1523-536X.2009.00378.x/full

Médecins Sans Frontières. (2008, April). Food aid basket missing critical ingredients—with dire consequences for children under two. MSF. Retrieved on August 16, 2011, from http://www.msf.ca/news-media/news/2008/04/food-aid-basket-missing-critical-ingredients/

Merritt, R.J., & Jenks, B.H. (2004). Safety of soy-based infant formulas containing isoflavones: The clinical evidence. *Journal of Nutrition, 134,* 1220S-1224S. Retrieved on August 16, 2011, from http://jn.nutrition.org/cgi/content/abstract/134/5/1220S

Miles, J., & Betts, M. (2010, September). Make infant formula hard to get says RMIT's Jennifer James. *Herald Sun*. Retrieved on August 16, 2011, from http://www.heraldsun.com.au/news/victoria/make-formula-hard-to-get-expert/story-e6frf7kx-1225928068723

Millennium. (2011). *Millennium Cohort Study*. Centre for Longitudinal Studies. London: University of London. Retrieved on August 16, 2011, from http://www.cls.ioe.ac.uk/text.asp?section=000100020001

Millington, D. (2011). Phytoestrogens & your baby. *Facebook*. Retrieved on August 31, 2011, from https://www.facebook.com/topic.php?uid=53828794953&topic=7548

Minchin, M. (1998a). *Breastfeeding matters: What we need to know about infant feeding* (4th rev. ed.). St. Kilda, Australia: Alma Publications.

Minchin, M. (1998b). *Artificial feeding: Risky for any baby*. St. Kilda, Australia: Alma Publications.

Mitchell, C. (2011, March). Challenge to Horizon Organic's DHA fortified milk. *Food Safety News*. Retrieved on August 16, 2011, from http://www.foodsafetynews.com/2011/03/challenge-to-horizon-organics-new-dha-fortified-milk/

Monbiot, G. (2007, June). Don't listen to what the rich world's leaders say - look at what they do. *The Guardian*. Retrieved on August 16, 2011, from http://www.guardian.co.uk/commentisfree/2007/jun/05/comment.g8?INTCMP=SRCH

Monteiro, C. (2011). The big issue is ultra-processing. 'Carbs'. The answer. *World Nutrition, 2,* 2, 86-97. Retrieved on August 23, 2011, from http://wphna.org/downloadsfeb2011/2011%20Feb%20WN4%20CAM5.pdf

Morrison, P. (2011). Breastfeeding after six months. In D.L. Michels (Ed.), *Breastfeeding annual international 2011*. Washington, D.C.: Platypus Media.

Mullaney, T.J. (1994, December). Martek sells its first product. *Baltimore Sun*. Retrieved on August 16, 2011, from http://articles.baltimoresun.com/1994-12-14/business/1994348144_1_martek-biotechnology-baby-formulas

Murano, P.S., Diep, C.S., Ettienne-Gittens, R., Girimaji, A., Spaulding, C., & McKyer, E.L.J. (2011, June). *TEXFAN UPDATE: WIC participants' consumption and feeding practices before and after the food package changes*. Paper presented at the Nutrition and Breastfeeding Conference: Growing with WIC, Austin, TX. Retrieved on August 24, 2011, from http://www.wicconference.com/wp-content/uploads/Murano_Peter-TEXFAN-Update-Handout-1.pdf

NCT (National Childbirth Trust). (2008, April). *NCT briefing: Formula feeding*. Retrieved on August 16, 2011, from http://www.nctpregnancyandbabycare.com/sites/default/files/related_documents/BF12%20Formula%20Feeding.pdf

NCT. (2010, June). *NCT briefing: The UK infant formula regulations.* Retrieved on August 16, 2011, from http://www.nctpregnancyandbabycare.com/sites/ default/files/related_documents/2BF7RegulationsonInfantFormula.pdf

NCT Watch. (2009). *Minister questioned about the inclusion of infant formula in Healthy Start.* London: National Childbirth Trust. Retrieved August 16, 2011, from http://nctwatch.wordpress.com/2009/03/27/minister-questioned-about-the-inclusion-of-infant-formula-in-healthy-start/

Nestle, M. (2006). *What to eat.* New York: North Point Press.

Neuberger, Z. (2010a). *WIC food package should be based on science: Foods with new functional ingredients should be provided only if they deliver health or nutritional benefits.* Washington, D.C.: Center on Budget and Policy Priorities. Retrieved on August 16, 2011, from http://www.cbpp.org/files/6-4-10fa.pdf

Neuberger, Z. (2010b, June). Podcast: New ingredients raising costs for "WIC" Program. Washington, D.C.: Center on Budget and Policy Priorities. Retrieved on August 16, 2011, from http://www.cbpp.org/cms/index. cfm?fa=view&id=3213

NICE. (2006). *Postnatal care: Routine postnatal care of women and their babies.* London: National Institute for Health and Clinical Excellence. Retrieved on August 16, 2011, from http://www.nice.org.uk/nicemedia/ live/10988/30155/30155.doc

Nommsen-Rivers, L.A. (2004). Does breastfeeding protect against infant mortality in the United States? *Journal of Human Lactation, 20*(3), 357-358.

Oddy, W.H. (2002). The impact of breast milk on infant and child health. *Breastfeeding Review, 10*(3), 5-18.

Oliveira, V., Prell, M., Smallwood, D., & Frazão, E. (2001). *Infant formula prices and availability: Final report to Congress.* Washington, D.C.: U. S. Department of Agriculture. Economic Research Service. Retrieved on August 16, 2011, from http://www.ers.usda.gov/publications/efan02001/efan02001.pdf

Oliveira, V., Frazão, E., & Smallwood, D. (2010). *Rising infant formula costs to the WIC Program: Recent trends in rebates and wholesale prices.* Washington, D.C.: U.S. Department of Agriculture. Retrieved on August 16, 2011, from http:// www.ers.usda.gov/Publications/ERR93/

Oliveira, V., Frazão, E., & Smallwood, D. (2011). *The Infant Formula Market: Consequences of a Change in the WIC Contract.* Washington, D.C.; U.S. Department of Agriculture. Retrieved on August 24, 2011, from http:// www.ers.usda.gov/Publications/ERR124/ERR124.pdf

Packard, V.S. (1982). *Human milk and infant formula.* New York: Academic Press.

Palmer, G. (2009, February). *The politics of breastfeeding: When breasts are bad for business.* London, U.K.: Pinter and Martin. Economic Research Report 93.

PCIJ (Philippine Center for Investigative Journalism). (2007, June). *The Philippine milk code: A timeline.* Retrieved on August 16, 2011, from http://www.pcij. org/blog/2007/06/20/the-philippine-milk-code-a-timeline/

PEDNSS. (2011). *Pediatric and pregnancy nutrition surveillance system.* Retrieved on August 16, 2011, from http://www.cdc.gov/pednss/

Pelletier, D.L. (2002). *Toward a common understanding of malnutrition: Assessing the contributions of the UNICEF framework.* New York and Washington, D.C.: UNICEF and World Bank. Retrieved on August 16, 2011, from http://www.tulane.edu/~internut/publications/WB_Bckgrd_Pprs/Narrative/NarrativeonePelletierfinal.doc

Petersen, M. (2003, December). Breastfeeding ads delayed by a dispute over content. *New York Times.* Retrieved on August 16, 2011, from http://query.nytimes.com/gst/fullpage.html?res=9A03E1DC173DF937A35751C1A9659C8B63

PR Newswire. (2011, April). *Emerald Dairy obtains AQSIQ certification on facilities and provides 2011 guidance.* Retrieved on August 16, 2011, from http://www.prnewswire.com/news-releases/emerald-dairy-obtains-aqsiq-certification-on-facilities-and-provides-2011-guidance-119173539.html

Probiotic.org. (2011). *Safety of probiotic products.* Retrieved on August 16, 2011, from http://www.probiotic.org/safety

Rabin, R. (2006, June). Breast-feed or else. *New York Times.* Retrieved on August 16, 2011, from http://www.nytimes.com/2006/06/13/health/13brea.html

Ramzy, A. (2010, August). Is tainted milk to blame for China's infant puberty? *Time.* Retrieved on August 16, 2011, from http://www.time.com/time/world/article/0,8599,2010044,00.html

Reis, S. (2011, March). Foods with health claims. *Nutraceuticals World.* Retrieved on August 16, 2011, from http://www.nutraceuticalsworld.com/contents/view/32013

Renfrew, M.J., Ansell, P., & Macleod, K.L. (2003). Formula feed preparation: Helping reduce the risks; a systematic review. *Archives of Disease in Childhood, 8*(1), 855-858. Retrieved on August 16, 2011, from http://adc.bmj.com/content/88/10/855.abstract

Reutersward, A.L. (2007). The new EC Regulation on nutrition and health claims on foods. *Scandinavian Journal of Food and Nutrition, 51*(3):100-106. Retrieved on August 16, 2011, from http://www.ncbi.nlm.nih.gov/pmc/articles/PMC2606979/

Richter, J. (2001). *Holding corporations accountable: Corporate conduct, international codes, and citizen action.* London: Zed Books.

Rosin, H. (2009). The case against breast-feeding. *Atlantic Monthly.* Retrieved on August 16, 2011, from http://www.theatlantic.com/magazine/archive/2009/04/the-case-against-breast-feeding/7311/

Ross, B., & Rackmill, J. (2004). *Milk money: Advocates say government pressured by formula companies to "water down" breast-feeding ads.* ABCNews.com June 4.

Rowlands, J.C., & Hoadley, J.E. (2006). FDA perspective on health claims for food labels. *Toxicology, 221,* 35-43.

Sarmiento, R.S. (2003, August). Wyeth products now free of GMO, says Greenpeace. *Philippines TODAY*. Retrieved on August 16, 2011, from http://www.bic.searca.org/news/2003/aug/phi/08.html

Schneider, A. (2010, May). Organized heists of meds and baby formula soar. *Huffington Post*. Retrieved on August 16, 2011, from http://www.aolnews. com/2010/05/10/organized-heists-of-meds-and-baby-formula-soar/

Shafai, T. (2009). Routine supplement of prebiotics and probiotics to newborn infants are not recommended [Letter]. *Pediatrics, 123,* e543-e544. Retrieved on August 16, 2011, from http://pediatrics.aappublications.org/cgi/ content/full/123/3/e543

Shubber, S. (1998). *The International Code of Marketing of Breast-Milk Substitutes.* The Hague: Kluwer.

Shubber, S. (2011). *The WHO International Code of Marketing of Breast-Milk Substitutes: History and analysis.*(2nd ed.). London, U.K.: Pinter & Martin.

Simmer K., Schulzke, S., & Patole, S. (2008). Longchain polyunsaturated fatty acid supplementation in preterm infants. *Cochrane Database of Systematic Reviews.* Retrieved on August 16, 2011, from http://www2.cochrane.org/ reviews/en/ab000375.html

Simmer K., Patole, S., & Rao, S.C. (2008). Longchain polyunsaturated fatty acid supplementation in infants born at term. *Cochrane Database of Systematic Reviews 2008*, Issue 1. Retrieved on August 16, 2011, from http://www2. cochrane.org/reviews/en/ab000376.html

Smith, J., & Ellwood, E. 2009. Feeding patterns and emotional care in breastfed infants. *Social Indicators Research.* doi:10.1007/s11205-010-9657-9.

Smith, J., & Harvey, P.J. (2011). Chronic disease and infant nutrition: is it significant to public health? *Public Health Nutrition, 14*(2), 279-289. doi:10.1017/S1368980010001953.

Sokol, E., Aquayo, V., & Clark, D. (2007). *Protecting breastfeeding in West and Central Africa: 25 Years implementing the International Code of Marketing of Breast-milk Substitutes.* UNICEF Regional Office for West and Central Africa. Retrieved on August 16, 2011, from http://www.unicef.org/wcaro/WCARO_Pub_ Breastfeeding.pdf

Stanner, S., & Smith, E. (2005). Breastfeeding: Early influences on later health. *Nutrition Bulletin, 30,* 94-102.

State of California. (2008, June). *Brown calls on CVS Pharmacy to end expired product sales, protect confidential information.* State of California Department of Justice, Office of the Attorney General. Retrieved on August 16, 2011, from http:// oag.ca.gov/news/press_release?id=1578

Stehlin, I. (1996, June). Infant formula: Second best but good enough. *FDA Consumer Magazine.* Washington, D.C.: U.S. Department of Health and Human Services, Food and Drug Administration. Retrieved on August 16, 2011, from http://babyparenting.about.com/cs/formulafeeding/a/formula. htm

The Economist. (2006, August). *The baby-food king*. Retrieved on August 16, 2011, from http://www.economist.com/node/7854488

The Economist. (2011, June). New Zealand's economy: Creaming along. Retrieved on August 16, 2011, from http://www.economist.com/node/18837157?story_id=18837157

Thorley, V. (2011). The dilemma of breast-milk feeding. *Breastfeeding Review, 19*(1), 5-7.

True, L. (2011, March). Letter to Glenis Willmott, Member of European Parliament. California WIC Association. Retrieved on August 16, 2011, from http://info.babymilkaction.org/sites/info.babymilkaction.org/files/CALWIC to GW.doc

Tuttle, C.R. (2000). An open letter to the WIC Program: The time has come to commit to breastfeeding. *Journal of Human Lactation, 16*(2), 99-103.

UBIC. (2010). Ingredients for the world infant formula market. *UBIC Consulting*. Retrieved on August 16, 2011, from http://www.ubic-consulting.com/template/fs/documents/Nutraceuticals/Ingredients-in-the-world-infant-formula-market.pdf

UNICEF. (2004). *Breastfeeding could save 1.3 million infants each year*. New York: United Nations Children's Fund. Retrieved on August 16, 2011, from http://www.unicef.org/nutrition/index_22657.html

UNICEF. (2007). *The milk code is for our children: Protect the milk code. Protect our children*. New York: United Nations Children's Fund. Retrieved on August 16, 2011, from http://www.unicef.org/philippines/RIRR-Supplement.pdf

UNICEF. (2011). *The Baby-Friendly Hospital Initiative*. New York: United Nations Children's Fund. Retrieved on August 16, 2011, from http://www.unicef.org/programme/breastfeeding/baby.htm

United Nations, Economic and Social Council. (1999). *Substantive issues arising in the implementation of the International Covenant on economic, social and cultural rights: General comment 12 (Twentieth Session, 1999) The Right to Adequate Food (art. 11)*. Geneva: ECOSOC E/C.12/1999/5. Retrieved on August 16, 2011, from www.unhchr.ch/tbs/doc.nsf/MasterFrameView/3d02758c707031d58025677f003b73b9?Opendocument

U.S. Centers for Disease Control and Prevention. (2010). *Breastfeeding*. Atlanta, Georgia: CDC. Retrieved on August 16, 2011, from http://www.cdc.gov/breastfeeding/

U.S. Code of Federal Regulations. Title 21 Part 106 (21CFR106). 2009. *Infant formula quality Control procedures*. Retrieved on August 16, 2011, from http://www.access.gpo.gov/nara/cfr/waisidx_09/21cfr106_09.html

U.S. Code of Federal Regulations. Title 21 Part 107 (21CFR107). (2003). *Infant formula*. Retrieved on August 16, 2011, from http://www.access.gpo.gov/nara/cfr/waisidx_03/21cfr107_03.html

U.S. Department of Agriculture, Food and Nutrition Service. (2010). Nutrition Assistance Programs Report. December 2010. Retrieved on August 16, 2011, from http://www.fns.usda.gov/pd/wicmain.htm

U.S. Department of Health and Human Services. (1985). *Guidelines concerning notification and testing of infant formulas.* Washington, D.C.: USDHHS, Food and Drug Administration, Center for Food Safety and Applied Nutrition. Retrieved on August 16, 2011, from http://www.fda.gov/ Food/GuidanceComplianceRegulatoryInformation/GuidanceDocuments/ InfantFormula/ucm169730.htm

U.S. Department of Health and Human Services. (2000). *HHS blueprint for action on breastfeeding.* Washington, D.C.: USDHHS. Office on Women's Health. Retrieved on August 16, 2011, from http://www.womenshealth.gov/pub/ hhs.cfm

U.S. Department of Health and Human Services. (2001a, May). *Agency response letter, GRAS notice no. GRN 000041.* Washington, D.C.: USDHHS. Food and Drug Administration. Retrieved on August 16, 2011, from http://www.fda. gov/Food/FoodIngredientsPackaging/GenerallyRecognizedasSafeGRAS/ GRASListings/ucm154126.htm

U.S. Department of Health and Human Services. (2001b, December). *Agency response letter, GRAS notice no. GRN 000080.* December 11. Washington, D.C.: USDHHS. Food and Drug Administration. Retrieved on August 16, 2011, from http://www.fda.gov/Food/FoodIngredientsPackaging/ GenerallyRecognizedasSafeGRAS/GRASListings/ucm154201.htm

U.S. Department of Health and Human Services. (2002, March). *Regulations and information on the manufacture and distribution of infant formula.* Washington, D.C.: USDHHS, Food and Drug Administration. Retrieved on August 16, 2011, from http://www.fda.gov/Food/FoodSafety/Product-SpecificInformation/ InfantFormula/GuidanceRegulatoryInformation/ucm136118.htm

U.S. Department of Health and Human Services. (2004a). *Infant formula: Overview.* Washington, D.C.: USDHHS. Food and Drug Administration. Retrieved on August 16, 2011, from http://www.fda.gov/Food/FoodSafety/Product-SpecificInformation/InfantFormula/default.htm

U.S. Department of Health and Human Services. (2004b). *Breastfeeding.* Washington, D. C.: USDHHS. National Women's Health Information Center. Retrieved on August 16, 2011, from http://www.womenshealth. gov/Breastfeeding/

U.S. Department of Health and Human Services. (2005). *How U.S. FDA's GRAS notification program works.* Washington, D.C.: USDHHS. Food and Drug Administration. Retrieved on August 16, 2011, from http://www.fda.gov/ Food/FoodIngredientsPackaging/GenerallyRecognizedasSafeGRAS/ ucm083022.htm

U.S. Department of Health and Human Services. (2009). *Notice to retailers: Sale of infant formula past the "use by" date.* Washington, D.C.: USDHHS. Food and Drug Administration. Retrieved on August 16, 2011, from http://www.fda.gov/Food/FoodSafety/Product-SpecificInformation/InfantFormula/GuidanceRegulatoryInformation/ucm106488.htm

U.S. Department of Health and Human Services. (2010a). Healthy people 2020 objectives – maternal, infant, and child health. *MICH-21-24.* Washington, D.C.: USDHHS. Retrieved on August 16, 2011, from http://www.healthypeople.gov/2020/topicsobjectives2020/objectiveslist.aspx?topicid=26

U.S. Department of Health and Human Services. (2010b). *Breastfeeding.* Washington, D.C.: USDHHS. National Women's Health Information Center. Retrieved on August 16, 2011, from http://www.womenshealth.gov/breastfeeding/index.cfm

U.S. Department of Health and Human Services. (2010c). *Beech-Nut Corporation 2/22/10. Warning letter.* Washington, D.C.:USDHHS. Food and Drug Administration. Retrieved on August 16, 2011, from http://www.fda.gov/iceci/enforcementactions/warningletters/ucm202834.htm

U.S. Department of Health and Human Services. (2011a). *Food safety. Product specific information – Infant formula.* Washington, D.C.: USDHHS. Food and Drug Administration. Retrieved on August 16, 2011, from http://www.fda.gov/Food/FoodSafety/Product-SpecificInformation/default.htm.

U.S. Department of Health and Human Services. (2011b). *The Surgeon General's call to action to support breastfeeding.* Washington, DC: USDHHS. Office of the Surgeon General. Retrieved on August 16, 2011, from http://www.surgeongeneral.gov/topics/breastfeeding/index.html.

U.S. Department of Health and Human Services. (2011c). *FDA 101: Infant formula.* Washington, D.C.: USDHHS. Food and Drug Administration. Retrieved on August 16, 2011, from http://www.fda.gov/ForConsumers/ConsumerUpdates/ucm048694.htm#NutritionalSpecifications

U.S. Department of Health and Human Services. (2011d). *Is it really FDA approved?* Washington, D.C.: USDHHS. Food and Drug Administration. Retrieved on August 23, 2011, from http://www.fda.gov/downloads/ForConsumers/ConsumerUpdates/UCM143301.pdf

U.S. Department of Health and Human Services. (2011e). *Infant Formula – Q&A.* Washington, D.C.: USDHHS. Food and Drug Administration. Retrieved on August 16, 2011, from http://www.fda.gov/Food/FoodSafety/Product-SpecificInformation/InfantFormula/ConsumerInformationAboutInfantFormula/ucm108079.htm

U.S. Department of Health and Human Services. (2011f). *Pathway to global product safety and quality.* Washington, D.C.: USDHHS. Food and Drug Administration. Retrieved on August 16, 2011, from http://www.fda.gov/AboutFDA/CentersOffices/OC/GlobalProductPathway/default.htm

U.S. Department of Health and Human Services. (2011g, April). *Letter to Deputy Administrator of National Organic Program, USDA.* Washington, D.C.: USDHHS, Food and Drug Administration. Retrieved on August 16, 2011, from http://www.ams.usda.gov/AMSv1.0/getfile?dDocName=STELPR DC5090415

U.S. Federal Register. (1996, July). *Current good manufacturing practice, quality control procedures, quality factors, notification requirements, and records and reports, for the production of infant formula, proposed rule.* U.S. Federal Register 61 FR 36153. Retrieved on August 16, 2011, from http://www.fda.gov/ Food/FoodSafety/Product-SpecificInformation/InfantFormula/ GuidanceRegulatoryInformation/RegulationsFederalRegisterDocuments/ ucm106557.htm

U.S. Federal Register. (2011, June). *Agency information collection activities; proposed collection; comment request; infant formula recall regulations.* U.S. Federal Register. Retrieved on August 16, 2011, from http://www.federalregister.gov/ articles/2011/06/07/2011-13941/agency-information-collection-activities-proposed-collection-comment-request-infant-formula-recall#p-13

Vallaeys, C. (2008). *Replacing mother – Imitating human breast milk in the laboratory.* Cornucopia, Wisconsin: Cornucopia Institute. (See website for updates.) Retrieved on August 16, 2011, from http://www.cornucopia.org/2008/01/ replacing-mother-infant-formula-report/

Vallaeys, C. (2010). *DHA and ARA in infant formula: Dangerous and unnecessary— Synthetic additives have no place in infant foods.* Cornucopia, Wisconsin: Cornucopia Institute. Retrieved on August 16, 2011, from http:// cornucopia.org/DHA/DHA-Update-2010.pdf

Victora, C.G., Smith, P.G., Vaughan, J.P., Nobre, L.C., Lombardi, C., Texeira, A.M., et al. (1989). Infant feeding and deaths due to diarrhea: A case control study. *American Journal of Epidemiology, 129,* 1032-1034. Retrieved on August 22, 2011, from http://whqlibdoc.who.int/hq/1993/44345_Article24.pdf

Walker, M. (2001). *Selling out mothers and babies: Marketing breast milk substitutes in the U.S.A.* Weston, Massachusetts: NABA REAL.

Walker, M. (2007). *Still selling out mothers and babies: Marketing of breast milk substitutes in the U.S.A.* Weston, Massachusetts: NABA REAL.

Waterfield, B. (2011, April). EU rules formula milk can claim it is as healthy as breastfeeding. *The Telegraph.* Retrieved on August 16, 2011, from http:// www.telegraph.co.uk/news/worldnews/europe/eu/8432808/EU-rules-formula-milk-can-claim-it-is-as-healthy-as-breast-feeding.html

Weimer, J. (2001). *The economic benefits of breastfeeding: A review and analysis.* Washington, D.C.: Food and Rural Economics Division, Economic Research Service, US Department of Agriculture. Retrieved on August 23, 2011, from http://ageconsearch.umn.edu/bitstream/33813/1/fa010013.pdf

Wellstart International. (2005). *Infant and young child feeding in emergency situations.* San Diego, California: Wellstart International. Retrieved on August 16, 2011, from http://www.wellstart.org/Infant_feeding_emergency.pdf

Whaley, S. E., McGregor, S., Jiang, L., Gomez, J., Harrison, G., & Jenks, E. (2010). A WIC-based intervention to prevent early childhood overweight. *Journal of Nutrition Education and Behavior, 42*(3S), S47-S51. Retrieved on August 16, 2011, from http://www.jneb.org/article/S1499-4046(10)00061-8/fulltext

Whitehouse, A.J.O., Robinson, M., Li, J., Oddy, W.H. (2011). Duration of breast feeding and language ability in middle childhood. *Pediatric and Perinatal Epidemiology, 25*(1), 44-52. Retrieved on August 16, 2011, from http://onlinelibrary.wiley.com/doi/10.1111/j.1365-3016.2010.01161.x/full

WIC (Special Supplemental Nutrition Program for Women, Infants, and Children). (2011a). Retrieved on August 16, 2011, from http://www.fns.usda.gov/wic/aboutwic/mission.htm Also see the WIC Briefing Room at http://www.ers.usda.gov/Briefing/WIC/

WIC (Special Supplemental Nutrition Program for Women, Infants, and Children). (2011b). *Women, infants, and children. Laws and regulations.* Retrieved on August 16, 2011, from http://www.fns.usda.gov/wic/lawsandregulations/default.htm

Wiessinger, D. 1996. Watch your language! *Journal of Human Lactation, 12*(1), 1-4.

Wikipedia. 2011. *Fonterra.* Retrieved on August 16, 2011, from http://en.wikipedia.org/wiki/Fonterra. (Also see *Sanlu Group* http://en.wikipedia.org/wiki/Sanlu_Group)

Willatts, P., Forsyth, J.S., Di Modugno, M.K., Varma, S., & Colvin, M. (1998). Effects of long-chain polyunsaturated fatty acids in infant formula on problem solving at 10 months of age. *Lancet, 352*(9129), 688-692. Retrieved on August 16, 2011, from http://download.thelancet.com/pdfs/journals/lancet/PIIS0140673697113745.pdf?id=4d037fefcb72946c:4d290c3d:12eee3be797:26eb1301082049056

Williams, C. (2005). *Breastfeeding and family foods: Loving and healthy.* Penang, Malaysia: World Alliance for Breastfeeding Action. Retrieved on August 16, 2011, from http://www.waba.org.my/whatwedo/wbw/wbw05/actionfolder.pdf

Witte, B. (2011, March). Md. governor to sign BPA ban in formula containers. *Bloomberg Businessweek.* Retrieved on August 16, 2011, from http://www.businessweek.com/ap/financialnews/D9M9K3BO0.htm

Wolf, J.H. (2003). Low breastfeeding rates and public health in the United States. *American Journal of Public Health,* 39(12), 2000-2010.

Women's Prison Association. (2009). *Mothers, infants and imprisonment: A national look at prison nurseries and community-based alternatives.* New York: WPA. Retrieved on August 16, 2011, from http://www.wpaonline.org/pdf/Mothers%20Infants%20and%20Imprisonment%202009.pdf

World Cancer. (2007). *Food, nutrition, physical activity, and the prevention of cancer: A global perspective*. Washington, D.C.: World Cancer Research Fund International.

World Food Programme. (2000). *Food and nutrition handbook*. Rome, Italy: WFP. Retrieved on August 16, 2011, from http://foodquality.wfp.org/FoodNutritionalQuality/WFPNutritionPolicy/tabid/362/Default.aspx?PageContentID=537

World Food Programme. (2010). *Fighting hunger worldwide: WFP annual report 2010*. Rome, Italy: World Food Programme. Retrieved on August 16, 2011, from http://home.wfp.org/stellent/groups/public/documents/communications/wfp220666.pdf

World Health Organization. (1981). *International code of marketing of breast-milk substitutes*. Geneva, Switzerland: WHO. Retrieved on August 16, 2011, from http://www.who.int/nutrition/publications/code_english.pdf. Also see subsequent related World Health Assembly Resolutions at http://www.ibfan.org/issue-international_code.html

World Health Organization. (2003). *Global strategy for infant and young child feeding*. Geneva, Switzerland: WHO. Retrieved on August 16, 2011, from http://www.who.int/nutrition/publications/infantfeeding/9241562218/en/index.html

World Health Organization. (2007a). *Evidence on the long-term effects of breastfeeding*. Geneva, Switzerland: WHO. Retrieved on August 16, 2011, from http://www.who.int/child_adolescent_health/documents/9241595230/en/index.html

World Health Organization. (2007b). *Infant and young child feeding in emergencies: Operational guidance for emergency relief staff and programme managers*. Geneva, Switzerland: WHO.

Young, A. (1998). A formula for danger: Selling of outdated infant food is widespread. *Detroit Free Press*. August 27.

Young, A. (2000). Outdated baby food sold despite danger. *Detroit Free Press*. April 7.

Zale, W. (2011). *Infant formula maker's ads about store brands barred*. The Financial. Trade Regulation Talk 2011-06-03. Retrieved on August 16, 2011, from http://traderegulation.blogspot.com/2011_06_01_archive.html

Appendix

Regulating Infant Formula

Issues:

- Government policy everywhere should recognize that poor health is more likely throughout the lifespan if infants' and young children's diets are based on formula feeding rather than breastfeeding.

- Safety standards for infant formula should be strengthened.

- Public policy should limit the exposure of children to excessive risk. Mothers should receive guidance to help them take risk considerations into account when deciding how to feed their children.

- Stronger measures should be taken to limit the use of outdated and counterfeit infant formula.

- Mothers should be advised regarding methods of feeding that are nurturing for the children. Where it is appropriate, rules should be established to ensure that agencies enable the nurturing relationship.

- The value of additives to infant formulas should be assessed through sound scientific procedures. They should not be assumed to be safe and effective.

- Standards for infant formula should require demonstration of nutritional adequacyade- as well as safety.

- Government agencies should limit the provision of infant formula or any other foods that place children at significant risk regarding their health.

- Procurement policies should be reviewed to ensure that they do not result in purchase of infant formula that is of questionable quality or overly costly to the government, program participants, or others outside the program.

- Regulations governing the ways in which infant formula is produced, marketed, and used should be strengthened at every level.

Examples of Failures in the System of Regulation of Infant Formula:

- Regulations have been based on the assumption that any formula for which the basic ingredients match up with a list of ingredients is *safe*, despite abundant evidence that the assumption is not correct.

- Regulations have been based on the assumption that any formula for which the basic ingredients match up with a list of ingredients is *nutritionally adequate*, despite abundant evidence that the assumption is not correct.

- Regulations are not based on systematic assessment of the effectiveness of each variety of infant formula in ensuring the healthy development of infants.

- Various additives to infant formula are assumed to be safe and effective, despite evidence to the contrary.

- Regulations are based on the assumption that formula will be used in an optimal way, despite the abundant evidence that it is not.

- The issue of water quality is ignored.

- Little effort has been made to provide clear information on risks, in a suitable form, to allow parents and policymakers to make well informed choices.

- There is no clear system in place to protect infants from outdated and recalled infant formula.

- Improper marketing of infant formula continues despite the clear guidelines in the *International Code of Marketing of Breast-Milk Substitutes*.

- Neither manufacturers nor governments undertake fair studies of the health and economic impacts of using infant formula to the extent they are needed to protect children's health.

- Government agencies provide infant formula at no cost, promoting its use, and thus undermine their campaigns to support breastfeeding.

From: Kent, G. (2011). Regulating infant formula. Amarillo, Texas: Hale Publishing.

Index

Author Bio

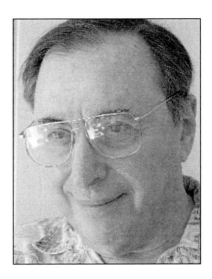

George Kent is Professor Emeritus with the University of Hawai'i. He was a professor in the Department of Political Science from 1970 until his retirement in 2010. He currently teaches online as a part-time faculty member with the Centre for Peace and Conflict Studies at the University of Sydney in Australia, and also with the Social Transformation Concentration at Saybrook University in San Francisco.

Professor Kent's approach centers on finding remedies for social problems, especially finding ways to strengthen the weak in the face of the strong. He works on human rights, international relations, peace, development, and environmental issues, with a special focus on nutrition and children. In addition to *Regulating Infant Formula*, his books include:

- *The Political Economy of Hunger: The Silent Holocaust.* New York: Praeger, 1984
- *The Politics of Children's Survival.* New York: Praeger, 1991
- *Children in the International Political Economy.* New York: Macmillan/St. Martin's, 1995
- *Freedom from Want: The Human Right to Adequate Food.* Washington, D.C.: Georgetown University Press, 2005
- (editor) *Global Obligations for the Right to Food.* Lanham, Maryland: Rowman & Littlefield, 2008
- *Ending Hunger Worldwide.* Boulder, Colorado: Paradigm Publishers, 2011

Professor Kent is Co-Convener of the Commission on International Human Rights of the International Peace Research Association. He has worked as a consultant with the Food and Agriculture Organization of the United Nations, the United Nations Children's Fund, and several civil society organizations. He is part of the Working Group on Nutrition, Ethics, and Human Rights of the United Nations System Standing Committee on Nutrition. His website is at http://www2.hawaii.edu/~kent

Ordering Information

Hale Publishing, L.P.
1712 N. Forest Street
Amarillo, Texas, USA 79106

8:00 am to 5:00 pm CST

Call » 806.376.9900
Toll free » 800.378.1317
Fax » 806.376.9901

Online Orders
www.ibreastfeeding.com